Training With Medicine Balls for Strength and Mobility

Guido Bruscia

TRAINING WITH MEDICINE BALLS FOR STRENGTH AND MOBILITY

40 FUNCTIONAL TRAINING EXERCISES TO BUILD MUSCLE AND STAY LIMBER

The Ultimate Functional Training Series, Volume III

Meyer & Meyer Sport

Original title: *Allenamento Funzionale - Manuale scientifico,*
© Guido Bruscia, 2013 Elika Srl Editrice via Fossalta 3895-47522 Cesena

Translation: AAA Translation, www.aaatranslation.com

British Library Cataloguing in Publication Data
A catalogue record for this book is available from the British Library

Training With Medicine Balls for Strength and Mobility
Maidenhead: Meyer & Meyer Sport (UK) Ltd., 2026
ISBN 978-1-78255-289-5

Aachen, Auckland, Beirut, Cairo, Cape Town, Dubai, Hägendorf, Hong Kong, Indianapolis, Maidenhead, Manila, New Dehli, Singapore, Sydney, Tehran, Vienna

Member of the World Sport Publishers' Association (WSPA), www.w-s-p-a.org

Printed by Print Consult GmbH, Munich, Germany
Printed in Slovakia

MIX
Paper | Supporting responsible forestry
FSC® C106855

CREDITS
Cover design: Kristina Ehrhardt, Anja Elsen
Cover photos: © Guido Bruscia
Photos: Chapter images on p. 18, 19, 32, 33, 35, 44, 45, 64, 80, 91, 111: Shutterstock (www.shutterstock.com)
Chapter graphics: © Thinkstock/iStock
The rights to all photos remain with the publisher
Layout: Kristina Ehrhardt, Anja Elsen
Typesetting: www.satzstudio-hilger.de
Copy editing: Elizabeth Evans

ISBN: 978-1-78255-289-5
Email: info@m-m-sports.com
www.thesportspublisher.com

Manufacturer under the GPSR
Meyer & Meyer Fachverlag und Buchhandel GmbH
Von-Coels-Str. 390
52080 Aachen, Germany
www.dersportverlag.de

CONTENTS

ACKNOWLEDGMENTS...

To my family, for never failing to embrace me.

To Ester, my partner and "muse", for our life together.

To my grandmother Sara, 106 years old, still functional today.

To Ernesto Rossi and Sabrina Parrello (and their children Ettore and Giovanni), for their great, true and unconditional friendship.

...AND THANKS

This book was born many years ago and is the work of the author and of all those who have been for him, even if unaware of it, a source of inspiration and ideas:

Emilio They (a friend and master never mourned enough), Marco Neri, Steve Cotter, Michael Boyle, Robert Dos Remedios, Alwin Cosgrove, Martin Rooney, Stuart McGill, Todd Durkin, Josh Henkin, Michol Dalcourt, Gray Cook, Marc Lebert, and many others who, for reasons of space (and memory!), I cannot mention.

Thank you also to all the friends, students, and colleagues who follow me with affection and respect.

Here, too, I can do justice to only a few of them:

Eda Maistrelli, Roberto Braghiroli, Claudio Arena, Emanuele Gollinucci, Roberto Cappelletti, my students at the Hamazon courses in Piombino and Castiglione della Pescaia, Bruno and Serena and the Mensana gym staff in Grosseto, Marco Giannoni and the Palestra Azzurra gym staff in Follonica, Mirko, and Cesare and the Living Club gym staff in Piombino.

Thanks also to the companies that help me with my work:

Elika Editrice

FitnessBest Innovation

Libertas

Ledraplastic

Tecnocomponent

Technogym

Newvitality

Superdry

Xconcept

Vibram Fivefingers

Vistawell

FOREWORD

Ever since humankind appeared on earth, people have always interacted with the environment in their own way.

Civilization has brought infinite advantages to the life of human beings but has also made them weaker and more imperceptive. The senses of smell, hearing and touch, proprioception, and the various organic capacities have all undergone modifications in the course of evolution from our ancestors to the present day. The result is that, while on the one hand we live in heated homes, on the other, a gust of wind is enough to send us to bed with a fever (Marlo Morgan, *E venne chiamata due cuori*).

Galen, one of the fathers of medicine (131-201 AD), wrote in his work *De sanitate tuenda:*

"...This is what I consider as physical exercise or gymnastics, a term connected with the gymnasium, where people go to anoint themselves, enjoy a massage, engage in wrestling, discus throwing or other sporting activities."

More than one thousand years after that, Mercurial recommended discus throwing, rope climbing, race walking, mountain climbing, and long jump as the activities that had the most benefits. People used to train with more or less rudimentary weights: medicine balls, dumbbells, rocks, the trapeze, ropes and still rings.

An athlete had to be strong, fast, and resilient.

Today, the immense popularity of gyms has produced centers which are extremely well-equipped, sophisticated, and multifunctional. Often, fitness centers imitate outdoor activities with much theatrical effect; they have free-climbing walls meant to resemble jagged, rocky cliffs, water courses and machines that mimic walking, running, and cycling outdoors. And yet, from many quarters, we see signs of a trend in the opposite direction: woodland programs, treetop walks in the woods, life-trails in parks, and a return to body-weight exercises, in which the body is the main training tool. The growing popularity of functional training is a sign that something is changing.

Worn down by the stress of urban life, people are returning to their origins; they are feeling the need for a stroll, a run, a different kind of muscular workout unconstrained by machines or showy equipment. They are looking for woods or meadows.

Nature all around, and, overhead, the sky as the only limit.

INTRODUCTION

When we talk about education, we refer to a system of knowledge which involves different fields of learning and is constantly evolving.

Gym activity requires the knowledge of physiology, anatomy, and biomechanics. Knowledge of nutrition and supplements also has proven to have an influence on sports performance and on results, and not just in terms of achievements. Also, in recent years, several studies have overturned many ideas and misconceptions connected with the world of sports.

Knowledge is an imperfect journey, full of trial and error. To these facts we have to add, of course, exercise practice, an empirical science which is by no means a given. Contrary to most beliefs, practice does not make us perfect: It is perfect practice that makes us perfect. The objective of education is to create professionalism, a word which, today like never before, plays a fundamental role in a coach's assessment. A professional is someone who provides a unique performance. Let's not forget this.

WARNING

This textbook has been written with the average fitness enthusiast in mind.

For this reason, I have glossed over issues which aren't strictly germane to the theme and sacrificed the purely technical definition of several concepts in favor of a more direct, straightforward language.

Medicalese doesn't help in assimilating concepts.

RESOLUTIONS

In 2004, at a personal trainers convention, I lectured on:

"Functional training for the lower limbs: A new perspective." In subsequent years, I studied the functional subject in depth, comparing my findings with those of several gurus in the USA, Spain, Switzerland, Germany, Slovenia, and Italy.

Functional training changes your life. Not your sporting life, which is focused on the search for optimal performance or, accordingly, for hypertrophy and super-toned bodies. Functional training simply makes people feel better, making them more active, stronger, tougher. In a few weeks, you will notice that your health is changing and that your physical efficiency and the well-being you are enjoying today have reached new heights. All this is the result of an optimization of factors which contribute to building a new body. It will not just be a matter of being more toned; there will be the awareness of feeling efficient for the first time.

Your body is like a custom-made outfit: It is the best place to live in.

All you have to do is try.

PART I – THEORY

CHAPTER 1

1.1 PRESENTATION

Every time we think about a sporting activity, we associate it with the concept of *motion*.

This process is so widespread and natural that we don't think about its underlying reason *why*. During courses, students who are interested in and passionate about training sometimes ask me why it is necessary to know stuff that has no apparent connection with a horizontal bench or a squat.

The answer is that gymnastics, in its broadest sense, is an empirical science; it stands apart from scientific bases which interact constantly with sporting exercise in gyms or outdoors. For this reason, you will often find not only various definitions, but also examples which refer back to practice.

The locomotor apparatus is the structure that allows a person to move in relation to space and the outside world. For practical purposes, it is subdivided into an active part and a passive part. The active part is made up of muscles, tendons, and ligaments. The inactive part is composed of bones and joints. Each is briefly discussed in the following sections.

1.1.1 The active part of the locomotor apparatus: Muscles, tendons, and ligaments

MUSCLES

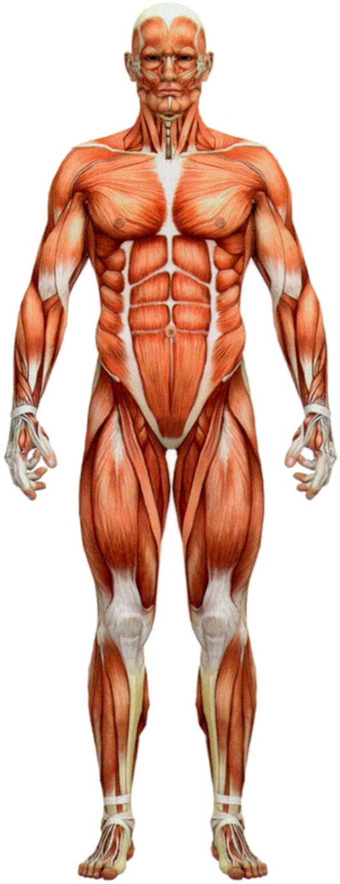

The term *muscle*, from the Latin *musculus* (from *mus*, rat, because some movements are reminiscent of a rat darting about), indicates an organ made of biological tissue with the ability to contract.

The muscles are subdivided into:

- Smooth, or involuntary, muscles
  Commanded by the autonomic nervous system, they encase the walls of several organs and corporeal systems, enabling or improving their functionality with their contraction.
- Striated skeletal, or voluntary, muscles
  Commanded by the central nervous system, they encase the skeleton, and, by their contraction (shortening), they determine the bone levers' movement.

A peculiar type of striated muscle is the myocardium, which is commanded by the autonomic nervous system.

TENDONS

Tendons are bands of connective tissue with poor elasticity, and their function is to anchor the muscles to the bones. Their role is to transmit tension from muscles to the bone levers, thus allowing their movement.

LIGAMENTS

Ligaments are sheaves of connective tissue with varying percentages of collagen fibers that link bones at the joints. The ligaments' purpose is to limit articular movement which would risk creating lesions were it to continue. For example, the knee's collateral medial and lateral ligaments support the anterior and posterior cruciate ligaments in limiting the articulation's intra- and extrarotation movements in order to avoid lesions to the knee itself.

1.1.2 The passive part of the locomotor apparatus: Bones and joints

BONES

Bones are specialized tissues with great mechanical resistance. They are divided into:

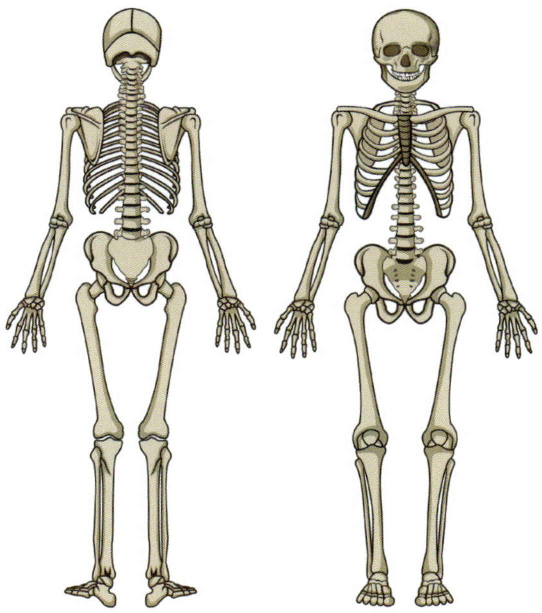

- Long bones (humerus, femur, tibia, radius): These are composed of an elongated body known as *diaphysis* and by terminal extremities known as *epiphysis*; they determine raw movements, which are characterized by wide articular excursions.
- Short bones (vertebrae): They have a similar diameter in all three spatial dimensions.
- Irregular bones (facial bones, the patella): These bones are characterized by variable dimensions and shape.
- Flat bones (pelvis, sternum, skull): Their function is protecting internal organs.

Don't be misled by bone tissue in the passive part of the locomotor apparatus: The bone is a highly active and dynamic tissue. In fact, from birth, the bone undergoes a remodeling process, involving the change and overlap of catabolic and anabolic phases. The catabolic phases are stimulated by micro organelles called *osteoclasts*, and the anabolic phases are activated by other specialized cells called *osteoblasts*. The piezoelectric effect gives the input for an increased bone tissue synthesis activity.

What does it involve? During motor activity, bone segment compression generates an electric depolarization of the bone membrane at the load points. This creates a greater localized need for the reconstructive osteoblasts. This explains why weight training, as demonstrated by several studies, has turned out to be an excellent remedy to contrast osteoporosis.

JOINTS

Joints are the junction hubs between two or more bone segments around which bones rotate.

According to their configuration and degree of mobility, joints can be classified as follows:

- **Synarthroses:** These are fixed, fibrous joints with little or no possibility of movement.
- **Amphiarthroses:** These joints are semi-mobile; they are often cartilaginous (e.g., vertebrae).
- **Diarthroses:** These are the mobile, synovial joints capable of a greater degree of movement. In terms of movement range, the most significant are the enarthroses (e.g., shoulder and hip), with spherical-shaped, multi-axial articular surfaces.

1.2 MUSCLE ACTION

For clarity, I have simplified the different muscular actions, adding the technical definition in parentheses.

- **Flexion:** When two bone segments move closer to each other (the moving part draws away from the horizontal plane). Example: brachial biceps, femoral biceps
- **Extension:** When two bone segments move away from each other (the moving part draws nearer to the horizontal plane). Example: brachial triceps, femoral quadriceps
- **Adduction:** When a bone segment draws closer to the median sagittal line (the moving part draws closer to the sagittal plane). Example: thigh adductors group
- **Abduction:** When a bone segment draws away from the median sagittal line (the moving plane draws away from the median sagittal plane). Examples: gluteus minimus and gluteus medius, high tensor fascia, deltoid
- **Torsion:** Movement of the trunk around the vertical axis.
- **Rotation:** Movement of a limb on its longitudinal axis.
- **Intrarotation:** Rotation of a bone segment in the medial direction, in other words, toward the inside (movement toward the anterior frontal plane).
- **Extrarotation:** Rotation of a bone segment in the lateral direction, in other words, toward the outside (movement toward the posterior frontal plane).

Each muscle performs several movements, which must be differentiated in order to better define exercises and their completion. For example, flexion and extension take place when the limbs aren't bearing weight. Bending, however, takes place when the limbs are bearing weight, as when completing a push-up. We may therefore notice that what is commonly referred to as flexing the arms is defined more correctly as bending the arms.

1.3 ROLE OF THE INDIVIDUAL MUSCLES

Based on the role they play in movement, we may differentiate muscles as:

- **Agonist muscles:** They play the main role in a specific action. Example: pectoral muscles in the horizontal bench press.
- **Antagonist muscles:** In the same action, they play an opposite role to the agonist muscles. Example: the trapezius muscle in the horizontal bench press.
- **Synergistic muscles** (from the Greek *sun-ergo*, "working together"): They help and support the agonist muscles. Examples: the triceps and anterior deltoid muscles in the horizontal bench press.
- **Neutralizing muscles** (stabilizers): They stabilize a bone segment, allowing other muscles to execute a certain action.
- **Fixator muscles:** They act as stabilizers, but they that is not their only role. They block a segment in the position that is appropriate to a movement or an action. Examples: pectoralis and latissimus dorsi muscles in parallel bars exercises.

1.4 ARTICULAR FEATURES OF MUSCLES

In gyms, muscle articulation is mostly disregarded, if not completely ignored.

Yet muscle articulation is of fundamental importance in understanding how to teach various exercise methods. Muscle articulation is defined as:

- **monoarticular,** those muscles that control only one joint and are inserted on bone levers that are paired by one joint only; and
- **bi- or multiarticular,** those muscles that cross over two or more joints.

In order to understand the importance of this distinction, let me remind you that when a muscle is biarticular, it should be stimulated with biarticular movements in order to be fully trained.

The most common example is that of the biceps brachii. Though it is a biarticular muscle, the biceps brachii is usually trained with monoarticular movements—the upper arm is kept steady against the trunk while only the forearm moves. To be clear, the monoarticular movement in this case isn't wrong, but it is nevertheless incomplete.

1.5 MUSCULAR TISSUE FEATURES

The features of muscular tissue are the following:

- **Contractility:** a muscle's ability to shorten.
- **Extensibility:** a muscle's ability to lengthen.
- **Elasticity:** the muscle tissue's ability to return to the initial length from a stretching position (the time factor needs to be evaluated, too).
- **Tonicity:** a very low-intensity electrical message which is always present within the muscle, even when at rest.

A common mistake is assuming that stretching helps only to elongate the muscle. In reality, there are many more effects of stretching:

- Extensibility
- Elasticity
- Articular flexibility
- Elongation of the connective tissue

For many years now, the concept of analytic stretching, in other words, stretching a single muscle or articular segment, has been surpassed in favor of systemic stretching, which involves longer muscular and articular chains.

More accurately, today we talk about mobilization, with reference to

- the joints, where muscles connect; and
- the connective tissue which covers the muscles and is less extensible than the joints; this means that when you talk about stretching a muscle, actually the range of the stretch is deeply influenced by the elasticity of the tissue that covers it.

1.6 ELEMENTS OF BIOMECHANICS: LEVERS

Biomechanics is the science that studies the law of mechanical actions in living systems.

Sports biomechanics studies a human being's movement within the process of physical exercise.

The study of biomechanics is essential when approaching any motor or sporting activity in order to identify

- the body's structure and motor functions; and
- the specific technique of the sport being studied.

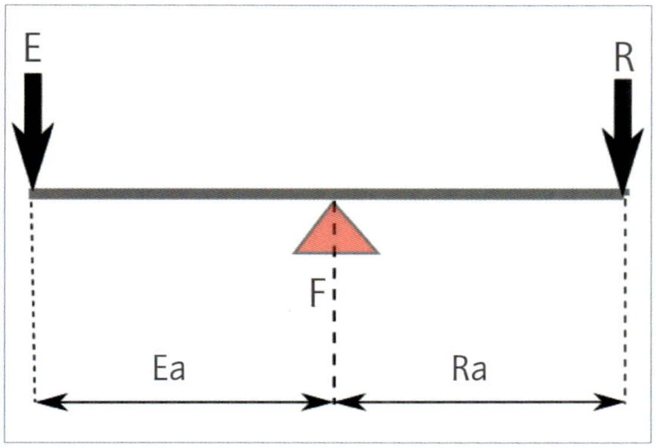

Lever in balance

A *lever* is a simple machine consisting of a rigid segment tied to a fixed point called a fulcrum (F), upon which two forces of equal strength but opposite direction are applied, called effort (E) and resistance (R).

The distance from the fulcrum to the point where resistance is applied is called the resistance arm (Ra); the distance from the fulcrum to the point where effort is applied is called the effort arm (Ea).

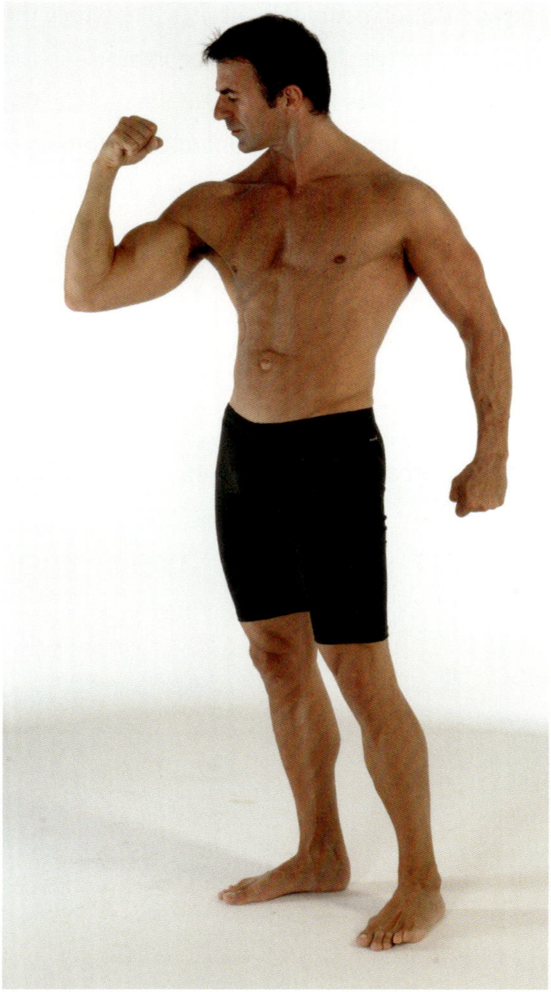

A lever is in balance when the resistance and effort arms are equal.

A lever is disadvantageous when the resistance arm is greater than the effort arm.

A lever is advantageous when the effort arm is greater than the resistance arm.

If we think about it, we realize that our skeletal system is a set of levers:

- Bones are the rigid segments.
- The fulcrum consists of the various joints that are involved.
- Resistance consists of the weight (load) we apply to the various levers.
- Effort consists of the muscles which contrast the weight's action.

The application point of resistance (i.e., where the resistance arm departs from) is the point of contact between the weight and the locomotor apparatus. The application point of effort (i.e., where the effort arm departs from) is where the muscle inserts into the bone segment. There are three types of levers in the human body, separated according to the distribution of the effort and resistance forces and the fulcrum around which the various bone segments hinge:

Type 1: Inter-fulcrum lever

The fulcrum is always positioned between effort and resistance. As we saw, a lever is advantageous, disadvantageous, or in balance according to whether the effort arm is greater than, smaller than, or equal to the resistance arm.

Example: a pair of scissors, a 45-degree calf exercise at the press machine.

TYPE 1 – INTER-FULCRUM LEVER

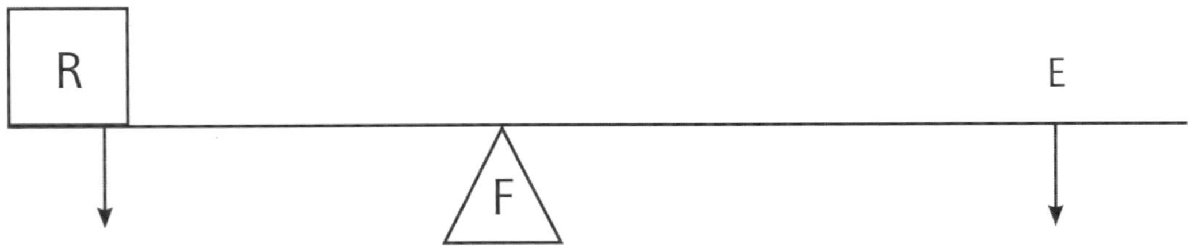

Can be advantageous or disadvantageous

Type 2: Inter-resistance lever

From its name we can deduce that resistance will always be positioned between the fulcrum and effort. The effort arm, therefore, is always greater than the resistance arm. The lever is always advantageous.

Example: nutcracker, standing calf raise exercise.

TYPE 2 – INTER-RESISTANCE LEVER

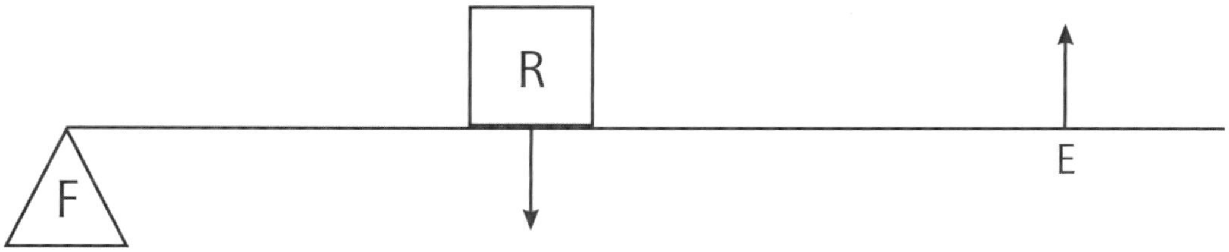

It is always advantageous!

Type 3: Inter-effort lever

The same logic applies: Effort will always be located between fulcrum and resistance. The resistance arm is always greater than the effort arm. The lever is disadvantageous.

Example: tweezers, biceps.

TYPE 3 – INTER-EFFORT LEVER

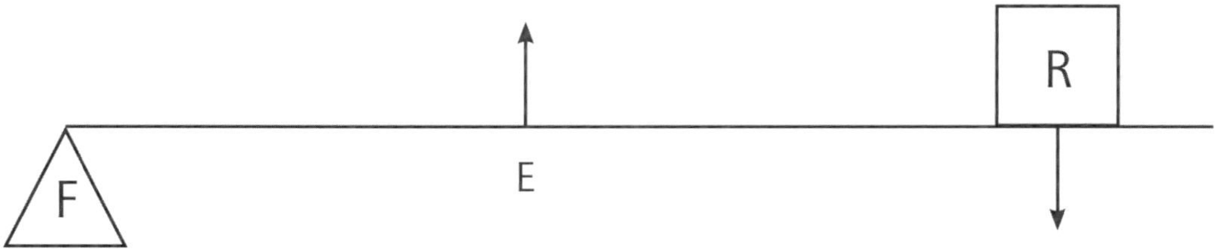

It is always disadvantageous!

1.6.1 Thoughts on organic levers

The majority of organic levers, at least when it comes to long bones (i.e., great locomotion), are type 3. Our body has opted for a predominance of disadvantageous levers. Why? Because this type of lever, though disadvantageous in terms of strength, allows wider movements and greater articular excursions and at high speeds. In practical terms, the evolutionary choice has been toward greater speed. (Let's keep these features in mind.)

CHAPTER 2

2.1 PRESENTATION

Life on Earth has evolved along the energy road, consuming energy economically and obtaining it easily. All living organisms now extinct (not because of human intervention) were inefficient energy systems and, as such, extremely wasteful. Living, making the body function, or performing any action requires energy. We can define *energy* as the ability to carry out a task. Specifically, a muscle is a chemodynamic machine; in other words, it functions through chemical reactions.

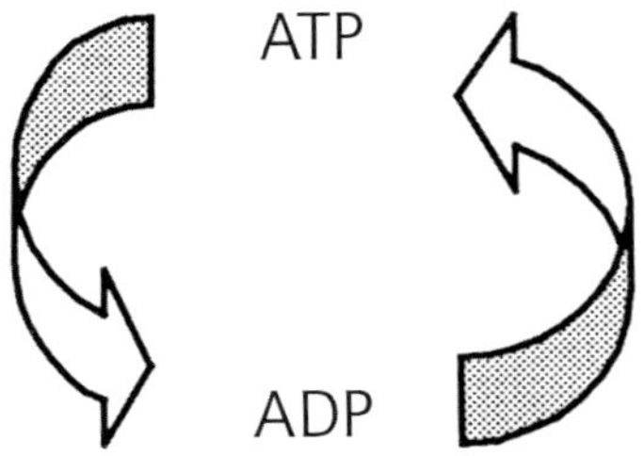

In order to convey a concept, it is useful to use imagery, visualizing the concept in pictures. To simplify the following chemical reaction, I will use imagery. Imagine a car. The model is called Man. Its fuel is adenosine triphosphate, or simply ATP. The human machine's universal fuel (its gasoline) is a molecule possessed of a high degree of chemical energy.

Our cells burn ATP continuously, and they are always synthesizing new ATP to obtain a supply of energy.

The gasoline's combustion in the car, Man, comes from the following reaction:

ATP → ATPase → ADP + P + Energy
Energy = (7.3 kcal/mole)

ATP breaks down into adenosine diphosphate, and this reaction produces energy.

The adenosine triphosphatase enzyme catalyzes the reaction (enzymes are substances which catalyze—they influence the speed of biochemical reactions, increasing or decreasing).

The amount of ATP present within cells allows them to work for a few seconds only. So how do they continue to work over time? They activate makeshift energy systems, with the objective of producing ATP (energy) according to the intensity and duration of the activity required. Intensity and duration cannot go hand in hand; they are two inversely proportional parameters. The more intensity (i.e., energy supply) required during an activity, the shorter the activity will be. Conversely, a lower intensity will allow a longer workout. Think about sprinting: You can run 100 m [109 yd] very fast, but you can't keep up the same speed to run, for example, 3,000 m [3,280 yd].

2.2 ANAEROBIC ALACTACID (CREATINE PHOSPHATE) SYSTEM

Let's imagine:

Car: Man
Model: Formula 1
Fuel: ATP + CP

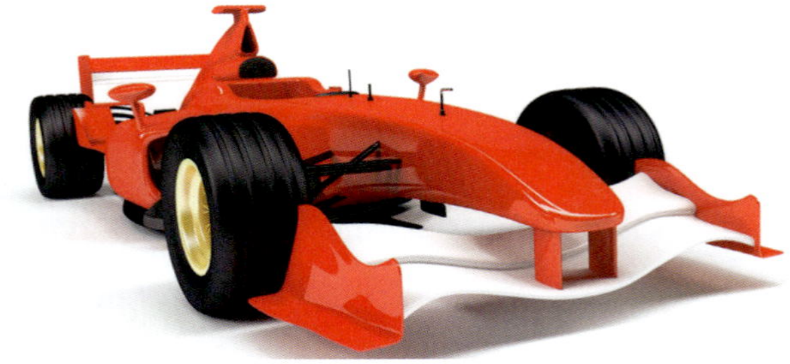

This system is used when an immediate supply of energy is needed for a very high-intensity but short-duration workout: 0-20 min (optimized at around 13 min).

What does the name tell us?

Anaerobic means there is no presence of oxygen; *alactacid* means that no lactic acid is produced.

We use a process called *phosphorylation:* The energy level of a substance is increased by binding it to a phosphoric group.

How is the energy supplied? Let's review the basic reaction:

ATP → ATPase → ADP + P + Energy

In this reaction, ATP breaks down into ADP. At this stage, ATP gets recharged by creatine phosphate (CP). CP doesn't supply energy directly, but it supports ADP, retransforming it into ATP, allowing the reaction to continue.

ADP + CP → cpkase → C + ATP
(Loehmann's mono-enzyme reaction)

The concentration of CP in the muscle is four to six times higher compared to that of ATP; this allows the energy supply to last a little longer compared to using ATP only.

Examples of sporting activities requiring CP for energy: 60-100 m [65.6-109 yd] sprint, long jump, high jump, strength training.

2.3 ANAEROBIC LACTACID SYSTEM

Let's imagine:

Car: Man
Model: Turbo-diesel sedan
Fuel: Glycogen/ATP

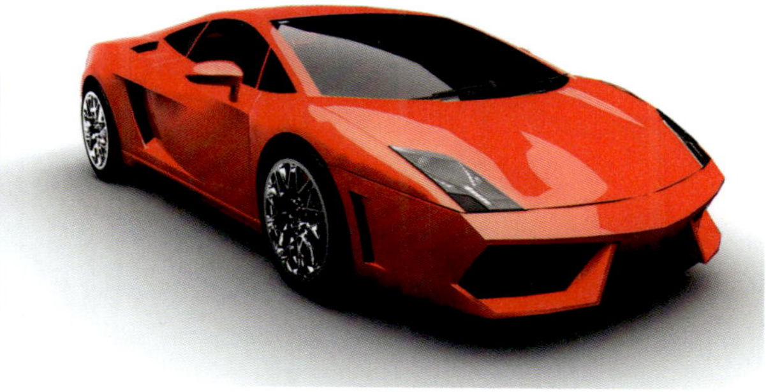

This system is used in performances that require a high energy supply for a medium-short duration. Let's analyze the name again. *Anaerobic* means in the absence of oxygen; *lactacid* means that there is lactic acid, or lactate, production. The ATP molecules are stored inside the muscles and the liver in the form of a complex sugar, an animal polysaccharide: glycogen (you can imagine diesel fuel). ATP is produced when glycogen breaks down into glucose, producing pyruvic acid and, subsequently, lactic acid.

This energy supply process is fast; it allows a high- to medium-intensity workout between 20 sec and 2 min (optimized around 30-40 sec).

The longer time required for the supply of energy compared to the anaerobic alactacid system is due to the 10 chemical reactions that lead to the breakdown of the molecules mentioned above.

Energy comes from the muscular glycogen and the hepatic glucose, according to the following steps:

GLUCOSE
↓
2 ATP
↓
PYRUVIC ACID
↓
LACTIC ACID

When one glucose molecule breaks down into pyruvic acid, two ATP molecules are formed.

This process is also known as *anaerobic glycolysis.*

This being a high-intensity activity with low utilization of oxygen, a highly acidic environment forms inside the muscles. Pyruvic acid binds to two excess H+ ions, producing lactic acid.

ADP + P + glucose ¨ ATP + lactic acid

When the lactate build-up becomes excessively high, the muscle's contractile capacity is inhibited (hypoxia).

What is the fate of lactic acid? Once the exercise is finished, it is partly used as fuel but it is chiefly re-converted into pyruvic acid and re-stocked in the muscles as muscular and hepatic glycogen (Cori's cycle).

Lactic acid isn't the cause for post-training pains!

2.4 AEROBIC SYSTEM (AEROBIC GLYCOLYSIS OR OXIDATIVE PHOSPHORYLATION IN MITOCHONDRIA)

Let's imagine:

Car: Man
Model: MPV car
Fuel: Macronutrients/ATP

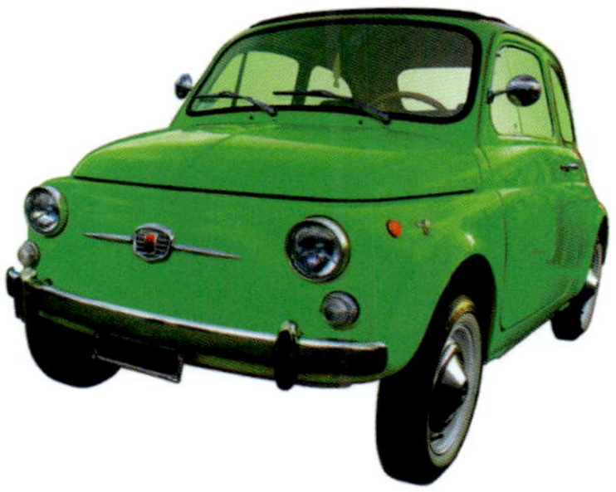

This system is used for all activities ranging from very low to medium intensity, lasting from a few minutes to some hours. Let's take a closer look.

Aerobic means the presence of oxygen is required.

Beyond the 2-min mark, only the presence of oxygen still allows glucose transformation; if the activity lasts longer than this, the system begins to activate processes which use stored fat as fuel. Compared to carbohydrates, lipids have a more unfavorable ratio between hydrogen and oxygen, and this explains the need to capture oxygen from outside to metabolize them. Proteins, too, provide energy within this system but in a lower percentage (3-5%).The process, also called *oxidative phosphorylation*, takes place within mitochondria, the cell's miniature power stations. The start is similar to the anaerobic lactacid system:

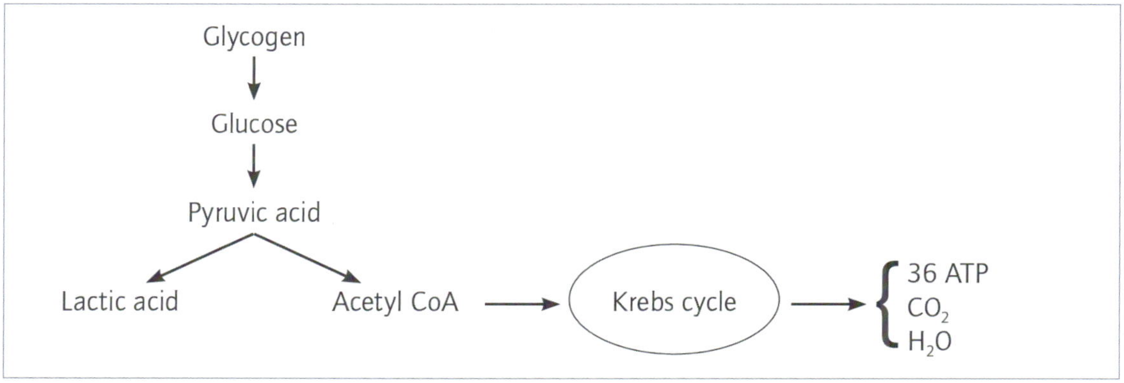

Because this is a reduced-intensity activity, pyruvic acid is transformed into acetyl-coenzyme A and transferred to the mitochondria, entering the Krebs cycle. The latter is like a metabolic furnace inside which the glucose molecule is completely broken down, generating 36 ATP, carbon dioxide, and water molecules.

In order to produce ATP, the aerobic system needs hydrogen. This is supplied by the Krebs cycle, exploiting oxidation (i.e., the removal of hydrogen) of food-derived compounds. Hydrogen is then transported to the respiratory chain via NAD (nicotinamide-nucleotide) and FAD (flavin adenine dinucleotide) up to the final receptor, oxygen, generating water.

Summarizing, the aerobic system is the result of two events:

1. Substrata breakdown, with production of hydrogen and carbon dioxide (Krebs cycle).
2. Hydrogen transportation to the respiratory chain, forming water.

2.5 ENERGY SYSTEM INTERACTIONS

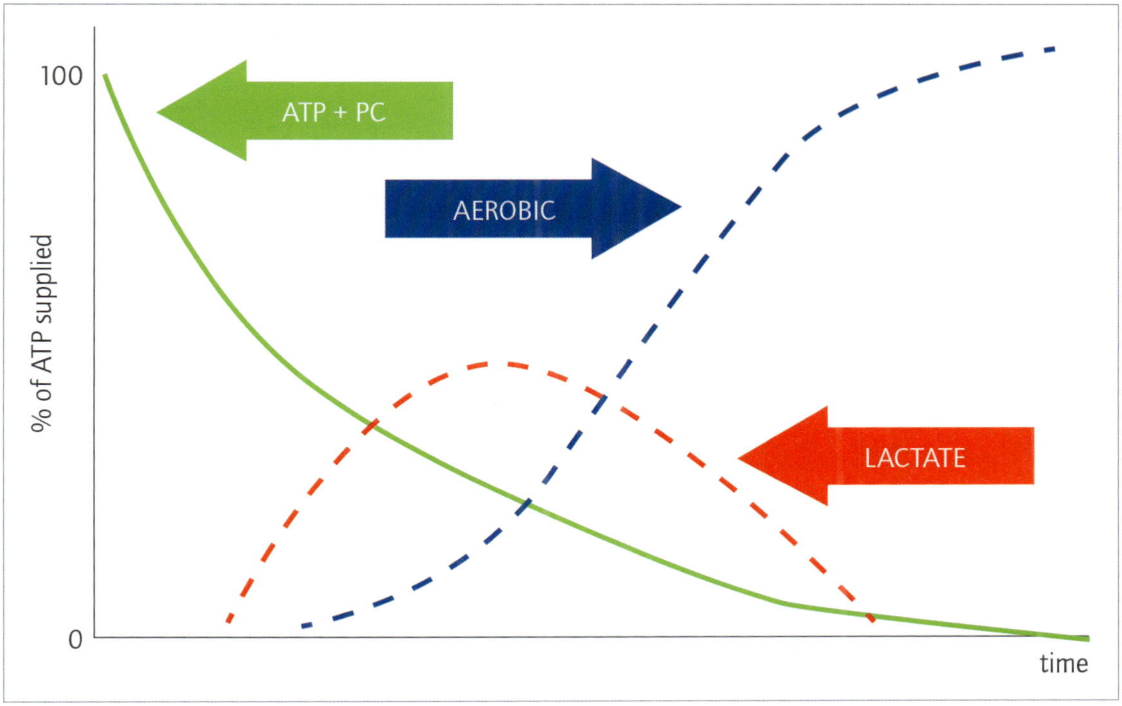

It is important to understand how the three energy systems cooperate.

The basic mechanism used by our body is the aerobic system. All the activities in our normal daily life take place at a low intensity and do not require a high amount of energy. This means that the aerobic system can comfortably provide the energy for all our daily activities. Whenever more intense efforts beyond the aerobic system's capacity are needed, the anaerobic systems work together with the aerobic system.

Note that in supplying energy, the three energy systems do not alternate like a relay. So when the synthesized ATP is active, it does not pass the baton to the anaerobic alactacid system, which in turn does not pass it to the anaerobic lactacid one. Instead, the three systems work together in parallel but also in different percentages, according to the type of effort, its duration, and the related demand for energy.

2.6 VO_2MAX AND THE ANAEROBIC THRESHOLD

The concepts connected to the terms *VO_2max, anaerobic threshold,* and *oxygen debt* are important.

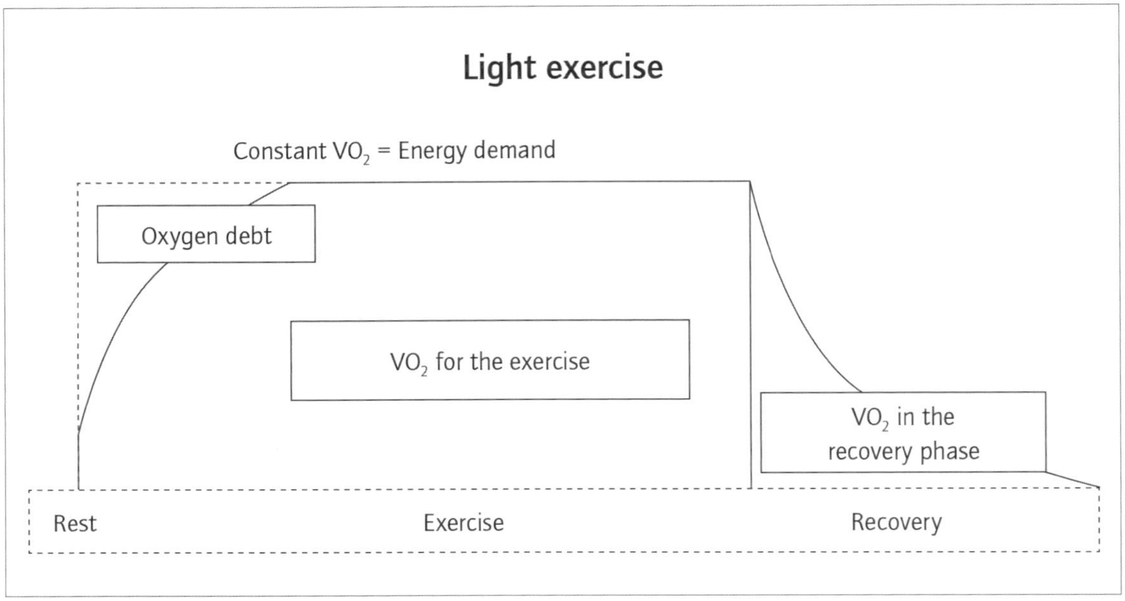

VO_2max, or maximum aerobic power, is in practical terms the organism's maximum capacity for synthesizing ATP using aerobics exclusively. It has actually been observed that this figure is more the result of a theoretical calculation than something reproducible in a lab or, even harder, in real life. An athlete is capable of maintaining an effort equal to VO_2max for no more than 10 min. Why? Besides a long list of factors—the majority of them genetic—the fact remains that at the experimental level it has been observed that well before reaching this limit the body begins to produce lactic acid. For this reason, at least in fitness training, the concept of anaerobic threshold has become increasingly important.

The **anaerobic threshold** is the maximum level of physical effort the organism can sustain without accumulating lactate in the blood. Above that heart rate the organism begins accumulating lactic acid because it cannot dispose of it as fast as it can produce it. The outcome is the fast onset of fatigue.

2.7 OXYGEN DEBT AND EPOC

Oxygen debt is the increased uptake of oxygen needed to remove excess lactic acid that is created by the increased synthesis of ATP which results from anaerobic physical exercise. What does this mean? We have seen that when you start a motor activity, there is an increase in the body's energy requirements. At the outset, the aerobic system isn't immediately available unless the activity is at a very low intensity.

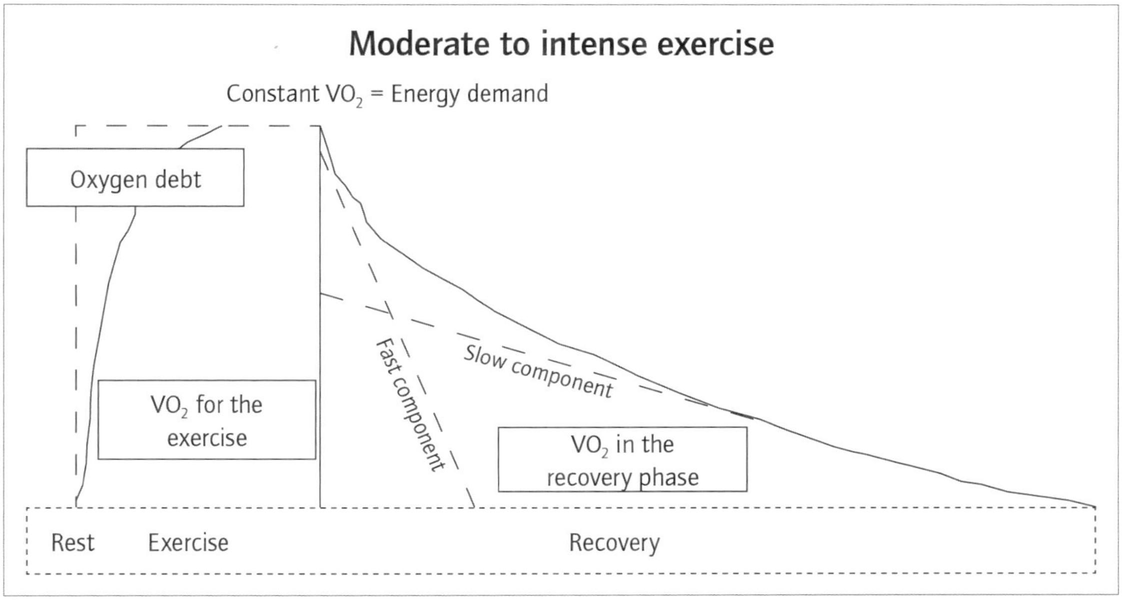

The body, therefore, requires help from the anaerobic systems, increasing the oxygen debt. The greater the intensity of the activity, the larger the debt. As soon as the effort is over, the body pays its debt by increasing oxygen uptake from the outside in order to restore phosphates and remove the lactic acid produced.

Dash or sprint for 20-30 sec. Now stop. What are you doing? You're panting. Your trunk leans forward, and your hands are on your knees. In order to increase your thoracic cavity's capacity, you inhale as much oxygen as possible from the air around you. This is the increased oxygen uptake.

Any exercise which involves the development of power above VO_2max is defined as *supramaximal*.

An oxygen debt can also be incurred as a result of a supramaximal load imposed on muscles; the oxidative machine intervenes in this case, too, at the end of the performance. However, in the ensuing recovery phase, the oxygen uptake exceeds the volume of the deficit. It's as though you're paying your debt with interest.

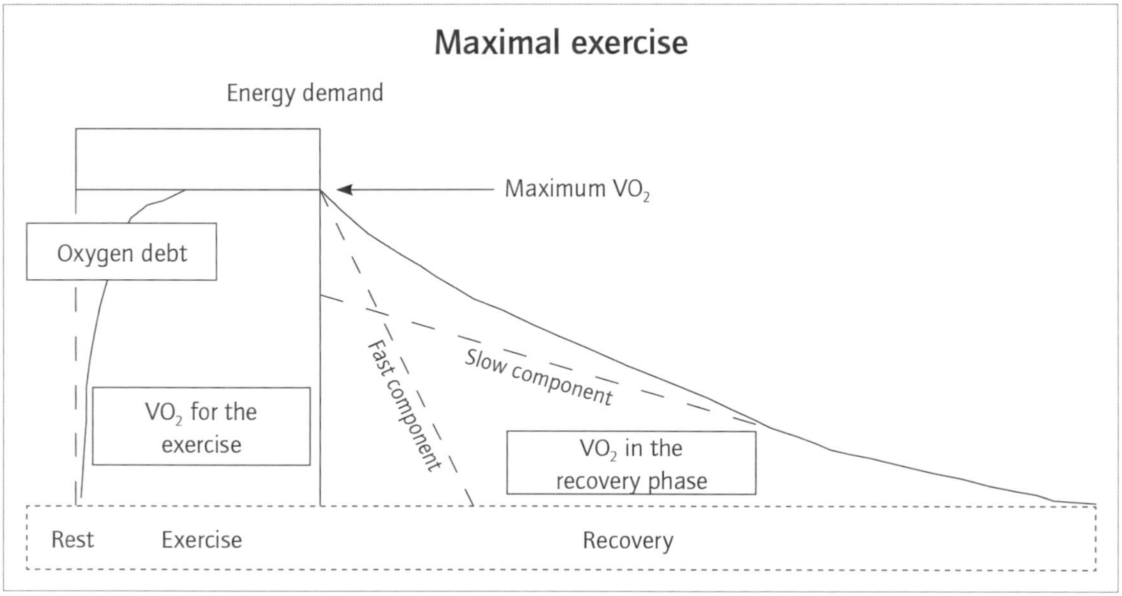

Margaria[1], R. (1938) has shown how the O_2 consumption curve during recovery can be split into four components:

1. **Constant component:** it depends on the subject's metabolism at rest.
2. **Fast component:** payment of the debt's alactacid fraction at a decreasing rate; lactate halves every 30 sec.
3. **Slow component:** payment of the lactacid debt at a slowly decreasing rate because of the energy cost of the renewed glycogen synthesis originating from lactic acid.
4. **Slow, long-lasting component:** attributed to the stimulus effect of the exercise on the metabolism at rest.

1 Margaria R. (1938). Sulla fisiologia e specialmente sul consumo energetico della marcia e della corsa a varia velocità ed inclinazione del terreno, in *Atti Accademia Nazionale dei Lincei* 7, 299-368.

With regards to this, studies show how the more intense a training session is, the higher the metabolism remains for a longer period of time in order to compensate the oxygen debt.

Recently, the concept of oxygen debt has been included in the wider concept of EPOC (excess post-exercise oxygen consumption). EPOC includes not just the oxygen debt but also the domino-effect adaptations which depend on it:

- Payment of the alactacid debt.
- Payment of the lactacid debt.
- Increased body temperature.
- Thermogenic effect caused by catecholamines.
- Renewed lactate synthesis.
- Renewed phosphagen synthesis.
- Lactate and blood oxygenation.
- High cardiac frequency.

CHAPTER 3

3.1 PRESENTATION

We have seen in the preceding chapters a presentation of the locomotor apparatus and of the energy systems through which the body acquires energy for movement.

Let's now focus our attention on the muscles, specifically on the processes which lead to muscular contraction and on the phenomena that result.

Let's introduce the main players:

1. The central nervous system (CNS). It consists of the brain, the cerebellum, and the spinal cord. From here voluntary muscular contraction originates through a nerve impulse.
2. The drive units. They consist of a body called *motor neuron*, an electric cable, the axon (including an insulating substance, the myelin sheath), and the muscular fibers stemming from it. The drive units' task is to carry the nerve impulse from the CNS to the muscle. The movement input reaches the muscle from the drive unit via a neurotransmitter (i.e., a substance which transmits a nerve impulse, called acetylcholine [Ach]).

3. The muscles. Each muscle is composed of a muscle belly surrounded by a sheath of connective tissue called *epimysium*.

- *Muscular fibers.* Inside the muscle there are groups of fibers bundled together in primary sheaths, or fascicles, encased by the perimysium. The primary sheaths are formed by muscular fibers encased by the epimysium; muscular fibers are in turn made of myofibrils, sheathed by the endomysium.

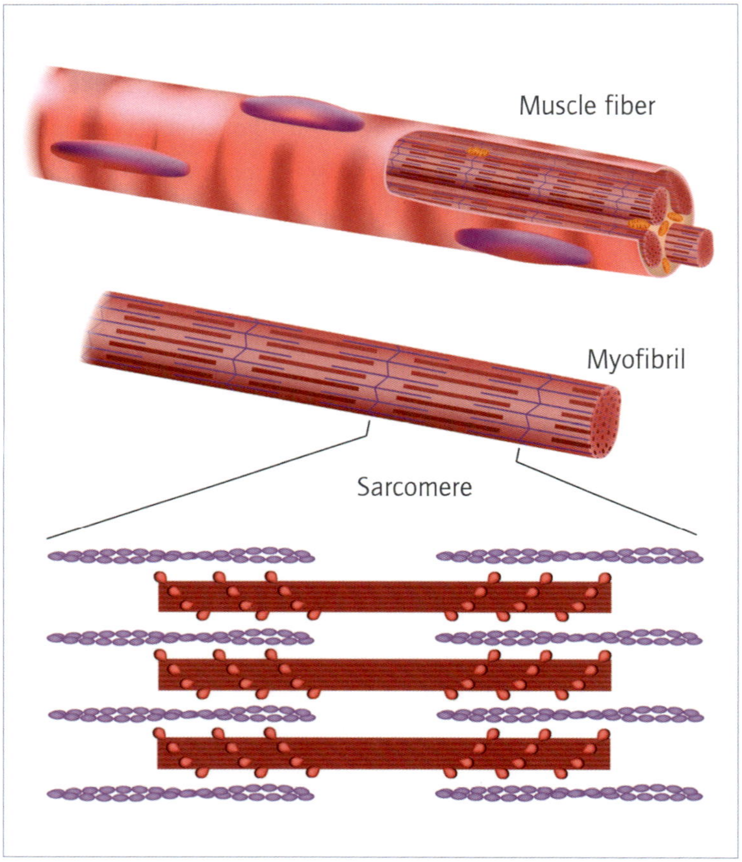

3.2 MUSCULAR CONTRACTION

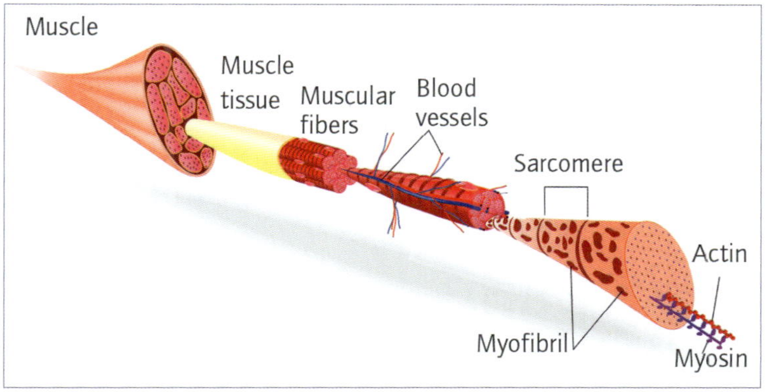

Skeletal muscle structure.

Viewed through an electron microscope, myofibrils appear as long filaments divided up into compartments by darker strips. Myofibrils can be compared with a train. The single cars, segmented by the Z lines, are called sarcomeres, and they constitute the cell's essential contractile unit. Inside each car (sarcomere) are two main regulatory proteins that partial overlap: actin (which is thinner) and myosin (larger, shaped like an oar or a golf club). We also find two other regulatory proteins, troponin and tropomyosin, interposed between the actin and myosin.

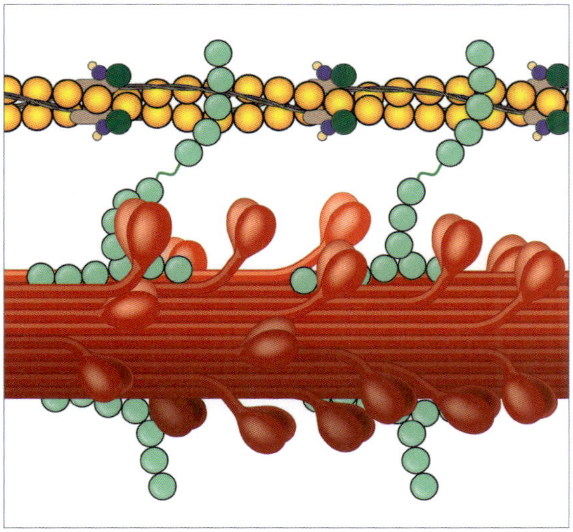

Actin and myosin.

Voluntary muscular contraction originates from the brain, goes through the cerebellum (movement is intermediary, making it fluid and coordinated), and reaches the spinal cord. From the spinal cord, the drive units incite the release of calcium ions from small cisterns called T-shaped tubules by releasing acetylcholine. The calcium ions bind with tropomyosin and troponin, canceling their inhibiting effect on actin and myosin. At this stage, the two main regulatory proteins come into contact. In the presence of ATP, the myosin heads attach to actin, pulling it and making it slide above them.

This sliding process is applied to every sarcomere inside the muscle and leads to its shortening or contraction (Huxley's myofilament sliding theory).

3.3 TYPES OF MUSCLE FIBERS

There exist two main types of muscular fibers, both possessing very different chemical and physical features.

- **Type I fibers,** or red fibers, or slow-twitch fibers.
  They are small and rich in mitochondria. They produce small tensions but are endowed with significant endurance.

- **Type II fibers,** or white fibers, or fast-twitch fibers.
  They are larger and produce high tensions but only for a short time. They hypertrophy very easily and are divided in two subgroups: type IIx and type IIa.

1. *Type IIx fibers* are known as pure white fibers and also as fast glycotic, with very few mitochondria, high tensile capacity and very limited endurance.
2. *Type IIa fibers,* or fast oxidative glycotic are also called intermediate fibers, since they share both some of the red and white fibers' characteristics: a good percentage of mitochondria, fine tensile capacity, and moderate endurance.

The percentage of fibers which innervate a specific muscle points to the type of training needed for it as well. For example, if hypertrophy is the objective, a muscle with a high percentage of white fibers will need to be trained with high weight loads, few repetitions, maximal or submaximal tensions, and long recovery periods. However, a muscle with a high percentage of red fibers will need to be trained with lighter weight loads, medium to high repetitions, and markedly submaximal tensions, though continuous and isotensive.

For this reason, the table indicating the statistical percentages of the various muscle fibers found within a muscle can provide excellent indications for a training program.

Table of the percentage of various fibers in some muscles.

Muscle	% STa*	% FTa*	% FTb*
Adductor brevis	45	15	40
Brachial biceps	50	-	50
Femoral biceps	65	10	25
Deltoid	60	-	40
Gastrocnemius	50	20	30
Gracilis	55	15	30
Adductor magnus	55	15	30
Latissimus dorsi	50	-	50
Gluteus maximus	50	20	30
Pectoralis major	42	-	58
Iliopsoas	50	-	50
Psoas	50	20	30
Rectus abdominis	46	-	54
Rectus femoris	45	15	40
Rhomboid	45	-	55
Semimembranosus	50	15	35
Soleus	75	15	10
Tensor fascia lata	70	10	20
Tibialis anterior	70	10	20
Trapezius	54	-	64
Brachial triceps	33	-	67
Vastus intermedius	50	15	35
Vastus lateralis	45	20	35
Vastus medialis	50	15	35

* STa = Slow-twitch fibres
FTA = Fast-twitch fibres
FTB = Fast-twitch fibres

3.4 TYPES OF MUSCULAR CONTRACTION

Muscular contraction is defined as the physiological means through which muscular fibers are recruited once the nerve impulse has arrived and given a sufficient amount of energy. Muscular contractions divide into two groups: static contractions and dynamic contractions. In static contractions the muscle doesn't modify its length, even though tension is developed. Dynamic contractions determine, on the other hand, a modification in the muscle's length.

1. **Static (isometric) contractions.** The muscle develops an amount of tension equal to the resistance applied, doesn't modify its length (the distance between muscular insertions is unchanged), and doesn't generate any output (in the physical sense, meaning there is no displacement). Isometric contractions may be
   - maximal: tension is applied with an unmovable load; or
   - stationary: the movement is voluntarily interrupted.

2. **Dynamic (non-isometric) contractions.** The muscle develops tension and changes its length, producing an output; the distance between the insertions changes during contraction. Non-isometric contractions may be:
   - concentric (positive): the tension developed is such as to overcome the applied tension; the muscle shortens, and the insertions draw closer.
   - eccentric (negative): the tension developed is less than the resistance applied; the muscle lengthens, the insertions draw farther.
   - Isotonic: the muscle shortens, developing a constant tension for the entire length of the shortening period. Actually, in reality, isotonic contractions do not exist. The tension developed varies as the lever varies. We can simulate isotonic contraction only with machines featuring physiological camshafts.
   - Isokinetic: the muscle generates the maximum amount of tension throughout the movement, shortening at constant speed (specific isokinetic equipment is used).
   - Auxotonic: the tension generated increases progressively as the muscle shortens (e.g., an elastic band).
   - Plyometric: explosive, concentric contractions immediately preceded by eccentric contractions; this exploits the energy accumulated within the muscle's elastic structures.

CHAPTER 4

4.1 ORGANIC SYSTEMS

Our body has 11 systems. Each system is made up of different organs. These 11 systems are responsible for complex physical functions. In other words, each system has a specific goal. The physical functions are:

PROTECTION

1. *Integumentary system:* the skin protects the underlying tissues, regulates body temperature, and synthesizes chemical substances and hormones.

SUPPORT AND MOVEMENT

1. *Skeletal system.*
2. *Muscular system.*

COMMUNICATIONS, CONTROL, AND INTEGRATION

1. *Nervous system:* it takes care of the generation, transmission, integration, and gathering of specialized nerve impulses.
2. *Endocrine system:* hormones are the main regulators of our metabolism, growth, development, reproduction, and other activities.

TRANSPORT AND DEFENSE

1. *Cardiovascular system.*
2. *Lymphatic system.*

TRANSFORMATION, REGULATION, AND MAINTENANCE

1. *Respiratory system.*
2. *Digestive system.*
3. *Urinary system:* kidneys cleanse waste from the blood. Inside the kidneys, the waste is transformed in urine.

REPRODUCTION AND GROWTH

1. *Reproductive system:* it guarantees the genetic code's survival.

All these systems exist in a state of equilibrium called homeostasis. The body constantly strives for equilibrium, reacting with negative feedback mechanisms to any sudden change.

Every time there is a sudden rise or fall in any system's parameters, the body activates certain physiological responses in order to bring the parameters back to the preexisting state of equilibrium.

Now, to avoid adopting the superior attitude of "experts" who train a different muscle group every day, you must understand that the stress applied on any system is also reflected on others and forces them to adapt.

Try this: Do a set of squats until you are exhausted. The effects? Respiration is fatigued, so therefore the cardiovascular and cardiorespiratory systems are stressed. The hip extensor chain—gluteus and quadriceps—is fatigued, and this means that the musculoskeletal system has been activated. Thighs and legs feel heavy, indicating the production of, the sign of an increased hormonal response (involving the endocrine system). We know also that among the physiological responses our body activates as a reaction to a stressful stimulus, such as training, there is an immune response. So another system is activated. Do you need to know more?

4.2 TRAINING: PRESENTATION

How to define training?

A person decides to start running, jumping, and doing push-ups with the arms and legs, doing this regularly until the onset of fatigue, trying to improve.

This means that this person is adding an extra energy stress (basal metabolism) to the daily energy consumption. This is not enough. This stress doesn't simply translate into greater energy consumption; it also translates into peripheral stress applied to the locomotor apparatus, which alters the equilibrium of the 11 organic systems that regulate this person's body. Sports training in physiology is defined as a stressor (i.e., a stressful stimulus). Compared to normal daily activities, stress is a series of factors that alter organic homeostasis, inducing a systemic response from the body. The systemic response is specific, depending on the type of stress involved, and non-specific, which is typical of all stress situations.

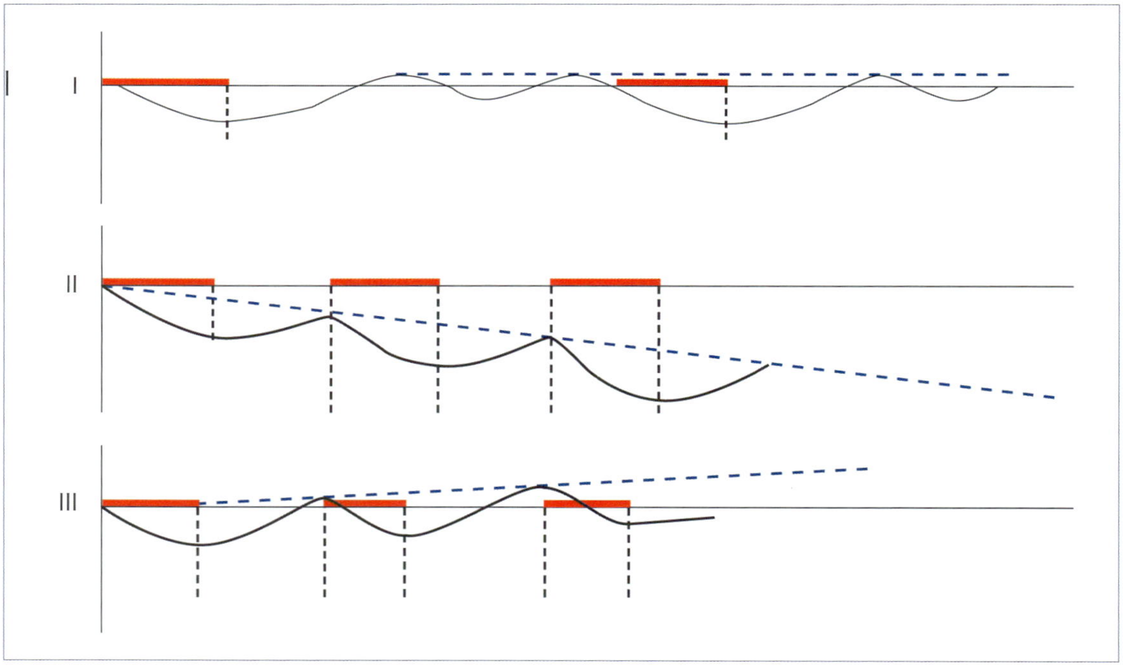

Selye's Law.

In order to be productive, stress must specifically have continuity (frequency), effort (intensity), and duration (volume). Training frequency determines the essential aspect that generates supercompensatory adaptations: recovery. This is what Selye's Law, or the law of supercompensation, says:

Following a stress situation, the organism activates a series of non-specific and specific responses involving the whole body, leading to a series of consequential adaptations after a suitable recovery.

The body effectively reacts to any stressful stimulus with a response and adaptation that are consequential and proportional to the stimulus received. Supercompensation will take place only after the organism has restored the conditions from before the onset of the training stress.

Improving a specific feature does not take place during the training session but during the following recovery phase; continuously subjecting someone to new training stress without allowing the body full recovery between sessions will cause overtraining syndrome (OTS).

4.3 TRAINING PROGRAM

Let's assume that training is the administration of stress, an additional burden to normal relational life that alters organic homeostasis in order to obtain a consequential response and adaptation (supercompensation).

In figure I (see section 4.2), the training stimulus is excessively rarefied.

This situation doesn't generate a chronic additional burden for the body, so there is no supercompensating adaptation.

In figure II, training stimuli which are excessively close to one another prevent supercompensating adaptation, quickly leading to overtraining.

In figure III, correctly scheduling training sessions over time leads to improvement.

You will notice in the definition of training the word *administration* is a pharmaceutical or medical term.

It was not chosen randomly. If training is to be scientific, its elaboration and training stimulus must be equally scientific.

Do remember: Each muscular structure has its own specific stimulus. This is a fact, even though it is true that certain stimuli, training for strength and its components, lead to improvement also in other structures, features, and characteristics.

Why? Any response is systemic: It involves the whole body.

Therefore a training program is the schedule of the stress (load) an individual must apply to his or her organic systems in order to obtain physiological modifications and related adaptations.

4.4 TRAINING THEORY

Let's now see which rules must be followed in order for training to yield results over time.

OVERLOAD

In order to induce physiological modifications leading to performance improvement, we must apply a training stimulus that is at least higher than that generated by normal daily life. This implies that once certain adaptations have been obtained, it will be necessary to train with workloads increasing in magnitude (load progressiveness) in order to further improve.

SPECIFICITY

A training stimulus will generate specific modifications in relation to the type of overload applied. Effectively, the benefits obtained from power training and those derived from aerobic training aren't interchangeable. In power training, we will have modifications typical of power training, while in aerobic training, there will be aerobic modifications.

INDIVIDUALITY

Given the multiple, infinite factors which differentiate one person from another, it isn't advisable to apply the same training program to all people, using identical stimuli, loads, and exercises. Training must be programmed according to the person , bearing in mind his or her physical, structural, and metabolic characteristics.

LOSS OF TRAINING

The effects of training are transitory and reversible proportional to the type, intensity, and duration of the applied stimulus. After 10-14 days of rest, there is a regression in several motor components already achieved.

4.5 TRAINING PARAMETERS

PLANNING

Plan training type and load rationally according to the amounts required by a specific discipline and by the goals to be reached in a well-defined time period. This takes place by structuring physical exercise in amounts and intensities that will provide progressively increasing workloads in order to stimulate the physiological processes of adaptation and supercompensation.

VOLUME

Volume represents the amount of work carried out during a workout unit. It is measured in different ways, according to the discipline referred to.

In bodybuilding, the total work volume is usually identified by the number of sets executed or the training session duration and by each muscle group's specific work volume (repetitions) or the time spent stimulating that same muscle.

INTENSITY

This is perhaps the most debated parameter and an object of disagreement between different schools of thought.

Definitions and formulas which are valid for performance sports aren't well suited to an anomalous discipline such as bodybuilding. In weight training, training intensity is directly related to the amount of kg [lb] lifted:

$$I = Kg\ [lb] \times R / T$$

I = Intensity
Kg [lb]= Kg [lb] lifted
R = Repetitions performed
T = Time needed to complete the set

This formula expresses a measure of power, since:

Kg [lb] x R

merely represents Work.

The work carried out in the Time unit expresses Power, but intensity isn't simply identifiable as the measure of the power output.

Intensity is the type of effort with which a certain gesture is carried out, implying a strong subjective component which is hard to measure.

- According to Prof. Emilio They, training intensity depends on the amount of motor units involved in the unit of time between a 0-degree and a 180-degree angle (extension) or between a 180-degree and a 0-degree angle (flexion).
- Intensity is a value related to the neurophysiologic mechanism of recruitment of the various motor units, and it is not necessarily related to weight, repetitions, and duration. It is therefore a personal and contingent factor which is not measurable through external data.

Intensity in a bodybuilding exercise is given by:

$$I = IC/N \times 100$$

I = Intensity
IC = Intensity coefficient
N = Total number of repetitions performed

While executing a set, you count the number of repetitions performed from the time when real fatigue sets in. This number is the Intensity coefficient (IC). When all is taken into account, the intensity parameter is probably the most important factor in training. There is a level of intensity below which there are no biological modifications inside the muscle; it is only a waste of time.

4.6 EXERCISES

Exercises are the means of training. They are the movements through which stress is administered by applying loads to the organic levers.

Choosing the correct exercises implies evaluating their effectiveness.

Let's distinguish between complex exercises, or general conditioning exercises, and competition exercises, or specific exercises (which reproduce a specific athletic movement). In athletic training, complex exercises are used to strengthen the whole locomotor apparatus, the conditioning abilities, and motor qualities.

Competition exercises instead reproduce or imitate the technically athletic gesture typical of a sporting performance. In physical education, this concept is simplified, and we prefer to differentiate between basic exercises and complementary exercises.

4.6.1 Complex exercises

FEATURES AND FUNCTIONS

- They are multiarticular.
- They work on long kinematic chains.
- They have great muscular synergy.
- They have a straight trajectory.
- There is greater external load (lifted weight).
- There is greater internal load (the external load's effects on the body).
- There is greater recruitment of motor units.
- It has great systemic response (endocrine, lymphatic, circulatory, immune).
- It is essential for ectomorphic subjects.
- It has great hormonal response.

RECOMMENDED USE

- In the initial stages of fitness training (the fundamentals).
- In the general conditioning phase, where they must make up at least 70% of the training elements.
- As strength mesocycles.
- As hypertrophy mesocycles.
- During the pre-competition phase, where they must make up at least 30% of the training elements.
- In slimming programs.

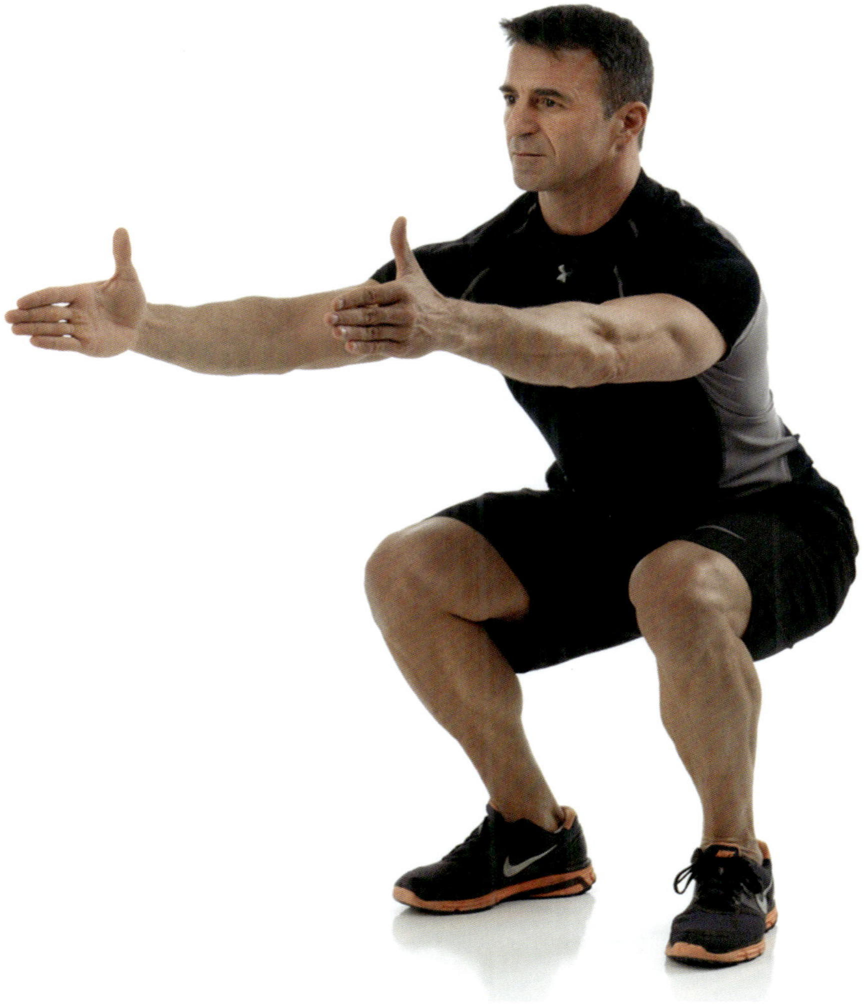

4.6.2 Competition exercises

FEATURES AND FUNCTIONS

- They are monoarticular.
- They generate a pinpointed, localized, targeted stimulus.
- They have low muscular synergy.
- There is a curved trajectory.
- There is greater muscular stretching (protein synthesis increases, both *in vivo* and *in vitro*).
- There is a lower hormonal response (a slight increase in GH).
- It has qualitative movement (i.e., correct, technical movements).
- It has low synergy.

RECOMMENDED USE

- In pre-competition phase.
- As hypertrophy mesocycles.
- In overload, high-intensity techniques.
- In highly sedentary, obese, or strongly overweight subjects.
- When working on specific areas.
- In postural training.
- In physical therapy training.

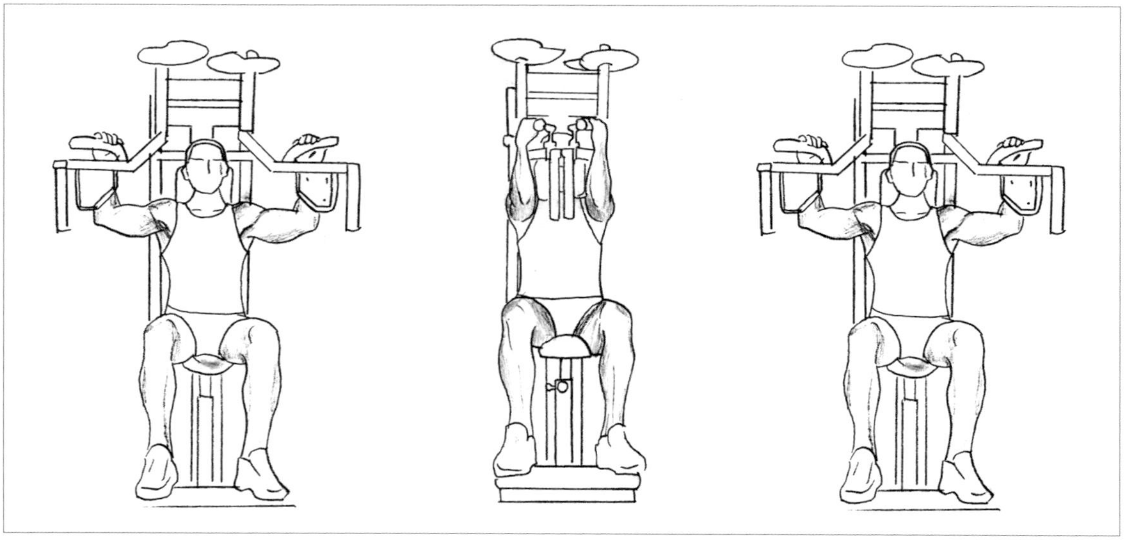

Given the high organic response they create, only basic exercises truly determine the greater effectiveness of a training program. Their prevailing factor is quantitative (i.e., the load). Complementary exercises have a mainly qualitative character, especially in the course of the specific training phase. In gyms, we must distinguish between, if you will, major league and minor league complementary exercises. Let me explain: In the weights room, we don't have a technical performance objective, and it is therefore important to concentrate on those complementary exercises which yield greater muscle stretching. Stretching, both in vivo and in vitro, can in fact increase protein synthesis and induce interesting adaptations.

CHAPTER 5

FUNCTIONAL TRAINING

5.1 KINETIC AND KINEMATIC CHAINS

In human articular physiology, monoarticular movements do not exist. We could perform them, but they aren't the priority for the locomotor apparatus. For economy and practicality, our body uses complex movements almost exclusively. In physics, *kinetic chain* is a system of rigid segments connected by mobile joints called junctions.

Our body is made up of many kinetic chains that are set off by our muscles. With the term *katakinetics* (Payr[1], 1936) or *kinematic chain* (Reuleux[2], 1934), we refer to the set of organs and systems that determine the human body's voluntary movements.

- By open *kinetic chain* we mean a system in which the furthermost end (the distal end) is free and unconstrained. Example: the lower limbs when walking.
- A closed *kinetic chain* is when the distal end is fixed. In other words, it cannot move during the execution of the gesture without involving another chain. Examples: squats or horizontal bench exercises.

1 Hanfried K. (2004). On the Development of the Constraint Motion Theory of Franz Reuleaux - An Overview, in *International Symposium on History of Machines and Mechanisms*, pp. 201-215.

2 Hanfried K. (2004). On the Development of the Constraint Motion Theory of Franz Reuleaux - An Overview, in *International Symposium on History of Machines and Mechanisms*, pp. 201-215.

5.2 THE MEANING OF FUNCTIONAL

The term *functional* is very trendy nowadays, with meanings ranging from A to Z. It's like an empty tube anyone can fill up as he or she pleases with everything and nothing. Our objective is to start with a scientific definition, without which it would be impossible to build a methodology.

Let's clear any misunderstandings by working with the dictionary definition.

From the Oxford English Dictionary, Functional: of or serving a function; designed or intended to; having a function.

You can't get any clearer...

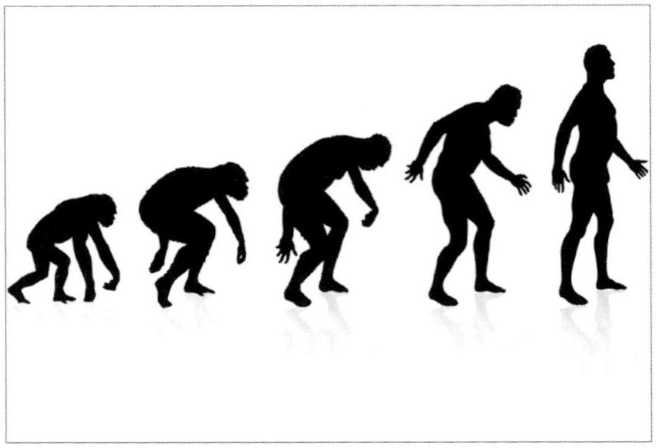

Functional training is a form of training that is related to the function for which a muscle, or rather a kinematic chain, exists and has evolved in a certain way.

The evolutionary choices of our locomotor apparatus explain the function of each muscle, kinematic chain, and articular system in our body.

How do we apply this concept?

a) by adapting it to each subject's articular structure.
b) by adapting it to the functions of the muscles or the kinematic chains which are activated.

The definition of functional training as training related to the function of the muscles in the course of a normal daily life isn't correct.

A reference parameter is actually missing: whose daily life? A weightlifting athlete's? A white-collar worker's? A sedentary person's? Daily life is different from person to person, but each one of us has the same kinematic chains.

5.3 THE ACTION-FUNCTION PRINCIPLE

The evolution in modern training is to train each muscle according to its action (a principle which is frequently applied in gyms) and to its function (a feature which is often neglected).

We must start by understanding the evolutionary choices of our locomotor apparatus.

Gyms have emphasized the concept of isolation to the extreme, focusing attention purely on muscular action but losing sight of the whole—the reason why that specific muscle, kinetic, or articular chain has evolved in a certain way.

From this stems the action-function principle:

The training of each motor feature or skill must be programmed on the basis of the action and function of the kinematic chain to which it is applied.

Without this type of programming, any training will inevitably be incomplete.

To simplify:

Functional training = Action + Function

For the same reason, functional exercises can hardly be defined as pectoralis, latissimus dorsi, or quadriceps exercises.

By working on kinematic chains as extensively as possible, large muscular areas will be engaged, even though one specific section will benefit the most.

The objective of functional training is systemic stress, involving as many organic systems as possible. This isn't enough. Understanding the evolutional changes which made us as we are today will help us understand how and why a specific muscle has developed a certain function and, consequently, how best to train it.

5.4 PEBBLES INTO A POND

Only by engaging the concept of functional training can we appreciate the shocking errors made in the development of exercises and methodologies which concentrate (often mistakenly) only on one aspect of training: action.

A few examples:

1. The femoral biceps and hamstring group

There are four muscular bands:

- Short end of the femoral biceps.
- Long end of the femoral biceps.
- Semimembranosus.
- Semitendinosus.

Of the four, only one is monoarticular: the short end of the femoral biceps. The action is flexing the lower leg to the thigh. The three others are biarticular, as they ride across the knee and hip joints. The actions are flexing the leg to the thigh and extending the thigh from the pelvis.

As stated in chapter 1, biarticular muscles must be stimulated with biarticular movements to be fully trained. In a gym there are no biarticular machines for the femoral biceps. Following the principles of biomechanics, training on the iconic leg curl machines, the only machines specific for this group, will always be incomplete.

Let's look into the function of the femoral group to discover which exercises will train it. For more information, refer to chapter 6 on the hip extensor chain.

2. The adductor group

The adductor group has three monoarticular bands and one biarticular one: the gracilis. The adductor's action is to adduct the lower limbs. The gracilis muscle adducts the thigh and flexes and medially turns the leg. The sartorius originates in the anterior part of the thigh; it is thus a part of the adductor group, but it acts synergistically with the gracilis (and with the femoral group, since it flexes the thigh to the pelvis), as flexor of the leg on the thigh.

In a gym these muscles are trained, especially in women, on the classic adductor machines. Let's think about it: Do we have our evolutionary choices in mind? Monkeys, from which we derive, all have the adductor group, yet we have never seen a monkey open and close its legs in any instance in daily life. It's evident that we have lost sight of this muscle group's function, and its training is therefore incomplete. What is the adductor group's function? The adductor is a muscle with the function of acting as a stabilizer; it's also a flexor and an extensor, according to the position of its contralateral limb. It must therefore be trained with multijoint movements, using body weight.

3. Abdominal fascia: The core

This is probably the worst-trained area in the history of weight training. In gyms, core training has become a saga: a thousand and one ways of doing crunches! As with the previous point: monkeys have the abdominal fascia, as we do, but do not perform crunch movements. It's clear, then, that the abdominal fascia has other functions besides the one we train with simple abdominal floor exercises. We must not forget we are bipeds and that our customary position is, or at least ought to be, standing. If we think about it, it is intuitive that the main function of the abdominal fascia cannot be that which is performed by exercising supine on the ground. We are now ready to answer these and other questions about functional training.

5.5 OBJECTIVES

The purpose of functional training is to totally develop conditional and motor skills and motor. In simple terms, we try to train an athlete who has a propensity for strength and endurance. In other words, this athlete displays hypertrophy that isn't purely aesthetic and disappears at the first cold, but it is functional. It is useful', so our locomotor apparatus will not easily do without it.

In addition, be defined as a strength and endurance athlete, an individual must have certain body composition parameters (unless the specific performance activity directs him or her toward different weight choices). Our athlete must therefore pay attention to nutrition and supplementation. He or she must also develop various coordination abilities, beginning with proprioception (perhaps the most important one), in order to prevent injuries and optimize performance.

5.5.1 What are the benefits of functional training?

Functional training is:

More adapted to organic physiology

a) it emphasizes the relationship between the locomotor apparatus and the environment.

b) in younger subjects and particularly in older ones, it optimizes the synthesis of vitamin D (the lack of which leads to an increased risk of fractures).

c) it allows all 11 endogenous systems to activate spontaneously.

d) it takes place mostly in the standing position. How often do we forget we are bipeds? And yet, statistically, we stand for only two hours a day. Presumably the bodyweight load at the lumbar level is the main cause of back aches.

More functional

a) because you do it standing up (an athlete always ought to train standing!).

b) because it activates long kinematic chains.

c) because it trains muscular chains according to the action-function combination.

d) because it trains all of the coordination skills.

e) because it follows our evolutionary history.

More effective for training compared to the classic indoor disciplines

a) in biomechanical terms.

b) in muscular terms.

c) in terms of the endogenous systems involved.

Let's just think about the difference between running on a treadmill and running on a road or dirt track.

In terms of muscular engagement, when running on a treadmill we do have the eccentric phase of the movement but the concentric phase—the extension of the thigh on the pelvis—is performed by the treadmill's own rotation, partially blocking the full motion of the gluteus. Furthermore, the foot strike is cushioned by the machine. The simple impact of the foot on the ground (not necessarily bumpy or unpaved) during a run or a walk outdoors has magnified consequences from a biomechanical point of view, and it also trains proprioception.

Also consider the work done using a road bike or a mountain bike compared to that done in a gym on vertical or horizontal stationary bikes.

5.6 MOTIVATIONS

The objective of functional training is to create athletes, forming our bodies into personalized outfits.

Another outcome of functional training makes it unique. Our motivation to become more fit on the outside goes hand in hand with improvements at the physical level. The more a person appreciates the progress and the strengthening of the organic systems (cardiorespiratory, endocrine, lymphatic, musculotendinous), the more that person will become mentally stronger, more determined, motivated and efficient. He or she will train in increasingly demanding conditions (rain, cold weather), with increasingly more intense activities (uphill and downhill running exercises, forest exercises).

Whoever said that functional, body-weight exercises are easy? Challenge yourselves on dirt tracks, beaches, meadows, or any other outdoor or indoor surface. Execute walking lunges for only 100 m (109.4 yd) because it doesn't matter how long you take; you can stop, rest, catch your breath...and then carry on!

Three days or a week later, return to the "scene of crime" and do the same exercise, but try one of three things differently:

1. Cover the same distance in a shorter time.
2. Take the same time but increase the distance covered.
3. Take less time and increase the distance.

Trying is believing!

5.7 FUNCTIONAL TRAINING AND PRE-ATHLETICISM

The term *pre-athleticism* can have two meanings:

1. Development of the athletic components in a child during the growth phase.
2. Training for specific performance sports.

And even a third new meaning, the one we refer to, about generic pre-athleticism or general physical preparation (GPP):

3. Multilateral work structured for the development of motor and coordinative abilities functional to a general psycho-physical enhancement.

In terms of this, Hirtz's[3] (1985) model identifies seven coordinative abilities:

1. Kinesthetic differentiation ability.
2. Movement combination and segmental coordination ability.
3. Reaction ability.
4. Orientation ability.
5. Balancing ability.
6. Adaptation and transformation ability.
7. Rhythmic ability.

To these general abilities we can add three others:

8. Motor learning ability.
9. Movement control ability.
10. Movement variation ability.

GPP work is, for the majority of athletes, the secret for working functionally and for wearing one's body like a dress.

Functional training will allow you to climb the steps of physical efficiency, while at the same time developing all those qualities which constitute the basis for it.

3 Hirtz P. (1985). *Coordination Abilities in School Sports*. Volk und Wissen.

5.8 FUNCTIONAL TRAINING: OTHER FACTORS TO DEVELOP

5.8.1 Training recruitment

Training recruitment means working on the central nervous system. The best age to obtain established improvements in this sense is before 14; specific training beyond this age will, however, improve several factors in recruitment, both spatial and temporal, though with a semi-automatic acquisition.

EXAMPLE 1

A child learns to ski and then, for whatever reason, doesn't practice this activity for a few years. When the child puts the skis back on, he or she will ski as well as before stopping (it will only be necessary to reacquire confidence).

EXAMPLE 2

An adult learns to ski with perseverance and frequency then, for whatever reason, doesn't practice for years. When the adult puts the skis back on, he or she will have to start almost from the beginning again (the stoppage time factor is significant).

Let's distinguish between spatial and temporal recruitment:

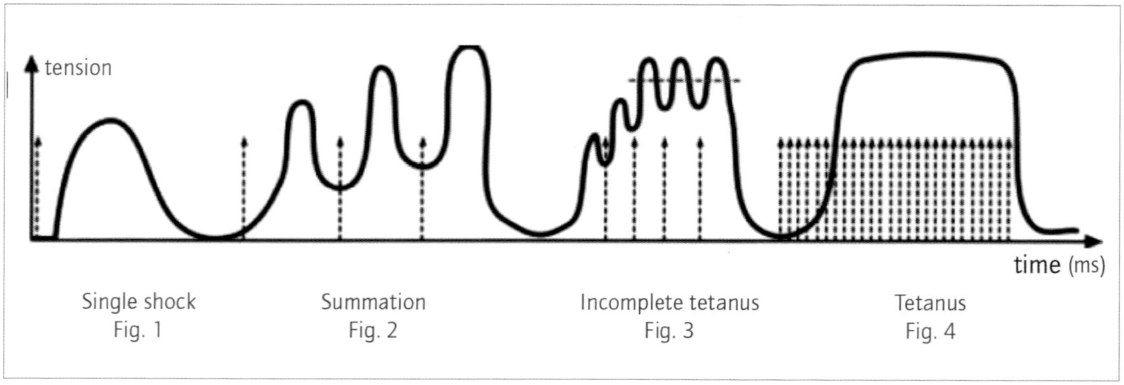

Summation

- **Spatial recruitment:** it is the increase in the number of motor units recruited during contraction and can be one of two types:

1. *progressive:* strength is developed gradually along the time scale (imagine pressing the foot down gradually on a car accelerator).
2. *ballistic:* the command signal reaches the muscle in a tiny window of approximately 100 ms (Paillard, 1982). Imagine flooring the accelerator immediately and hard.

- **Temporal recruitment:** it's the increase in the discharge frequency by the nervous system (via summation).

  - When a motor signal is sent by the central nervous system to a single fiber, the fiber first contracts then releases (fig. 1).
  - When the motor message is transmitted more effectively by increasing the impulse frequency, the tension generated by the muscle increases through the summation effect of two closely-spaced impulses (fig. 2).
  - With several closely-spaced impulses, the tension produced will increase further as a result of their summation, the clonus condition (fig. 3).
  - Beyond this limit, if the impulse frequency increases still, the maximum possible tension, called the tetanus, is developed (fig. 4).

5.8.1.1 Training recruitment in adults

It is possible to train the central nervous system, hence training recruitment, in adults. The objective is to increase neuromuscular activation by performing exercises outside the usual criteria:

- **More complex exercises:** involving long chains and working with several body districts together in order to force the central nervous system to engage in a higher effort.
- *Uncomfortable, destabilizing exercises:* using unconventional or differentiated equipment, making the execution more difficult; working from a standing position with differentiated loads, involving the body's stabilizing systems and muscles.

- **Plyometric and isometric contractions:** alternate to the normal concentric and eccentric phases. Varying the type of contraction within the same exercise has an uncommon training impact.
- **Working on the muscle's elastic components:** with exercises which involve a pre-stretching of the muscle trained (i.e., pulling away its origin and insertion). We forget that working with these factors is inside us—it is part of primitive activities such as running, walking, jumping, and sprinting.
- **Functional exercises:** training the muscles according to the action-function principle.

5.8.2 Strengthening pivot muscles

Whatever its objectives, training must reinforce pivot muscles for preventative and also performance improvement purposes. By pivot we mean those muscle groups belonging mainly to the deep musculature with the main function of joint stabilization—muscles which are loaded with tension during exercise performance.

The main ones are:

- Rotator cuff
- Flexors and extensors of the forearm and fingers
- Periscapular muscles
- Wide abdominal muscles
- Paravertebral muscles
- Tibial and adductor muscles
- Triceps surae muscle

When building an athlete, training these groups must take precedence over training others.

5.8.3 Reinforcing the weak links in the kinematic chains

It is of utmost importance when training to remember in a kinematic chain, the weakest muscle influences the functionality of the entire chain. If we have a chain made of several iron links and one paper link, the paper link will be the first to give way, and because of its frailty, will weaken the whole chain. Working on kinematic chains allows us to examine the weakest muscular links and to work on strengthening them using

- chains,
- elastics bands,
- kettlebells,
- sandbags,
- medicine balls, and
- shortened movements with supports.

Contrary to common wisdom, work on the weak link should not be aimed at hypertrophy. We must always take into account the synergy of the muscles involved in the same chain.

5.8.4 Breaking the pattern

This is one of the most interesting aspects of functional training: the ability to progress in a thousand different directions, to apply a variety of stimuli which gym activity cannot provide. Any structure, any object, whether natural or not—a tree, a branch, a rock, a rising slope, a flight of steps, a sand or cement sack, a wood, a beach, a track, a meadow, a dirt track, a low wall—can become the center of new workouts, new exercises, or new applications of the same.

The first step in breaking the pattern and building a motor map as wide as possible is to stimulate the central nervous system with basic exercise programs and unconventional exercises—the key principle being movement variation. And change an exercise not session by session but set by set, within the same session.

Every time we subject our central nervous system (and consequently the locomotor apparatus) to a new type of movement, we apply stress to it. At this stage, the central nervous system will be forced to adapt and enhance all the systems involved, owing to the continuity and repetition of the movement. A body which is prodded by multiple stimuli will be always proactive, ready to change; it will be able to react and adapt much more quickly. Variability of movement is the central nervous system's oil (Guido Veestagen[4], 2014).

As an example of what we mean, let's describe an exercise and its progression set by set:

1. Walking lunge.
2. Asymmetric walking lunge (weight on one arm only).
3. Walking lunge with two dumbbells.
4. Overhead walking lunge (one arm lifts the weight above the head).

Working on long kinematic chains, for example, is almost unknown in gyms, excepting squats and deadlifts. These are typical weightlifting technical gestures in which, after the loading phase, the weight is heaved upward and the body is simultaneously lowered in the opposite direction, fitting underneath the load. They are extremely difficult for the average gym patron, who is used to heavy loads but extremely simple exercises.

4 Veestagen G., (2010-2012-2014). Personal communication, *Perform Better Convention*, LA.

CHAPTER 6

6.1 PRESENTATION

Ask any athletics coach from Eastern European countries or the US: "Where does the secret of strength lie? Where does it come from?" They will reply: "From the hips, from the hip extensor chain". Hip muscles express strength and power more so than other muscles. It is not a coincidence part of the hip extensor chain is the gluteus, the human body's strongest muscle (after the masseter, the chewing muscle). Think of any performance sport and you will see that in some way this chain is deeply involved in it.

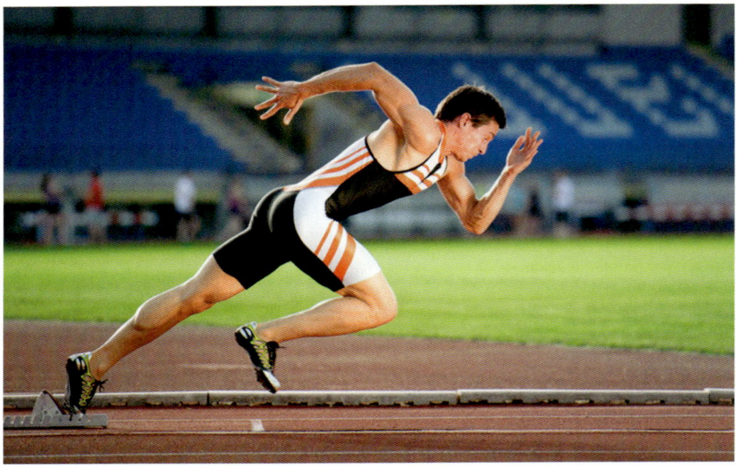

Training the lower limbs has a great importance in terms of prevention and pre-athleticism, even more than aesthetics. Studies provide ample confirmation of this when training is supported by basic exercises. Let's start with what we know: Ample articular excursions in the lower limbs (i.e., full squats) determine significant hormonal distress (Bosco[1] and coll., 1996).

It is clear then: the lower limb training bastions (squats, leg presses, sagittal lunges, deadlifts) do work. Their combined use satisfies any and all needs for strength, tone, and muscular tropism. But the question we must ask ourselves is: do they train thighs and glutes completely? The answer is no! These exercises actually train the gluteus, the quadriceps, and in general the lower limb muscles according to their action and the flexion and extension of the thigh on the pelvis, but not their function.

Do we remember the concept of functional training? It is Action + Function. What is the function of the gluteus? It is propulsion.

Now take a look around gyms, and you will notice that there are no exercises featuring propulsion or that work with propulsion in any way.

In the training this chain, exercises in which this thrusting action is present are missing, such as

- jumps,
- skips,.
- plyometric jumps,
- uphill walking,
- sprinting (better if uphill),
- starter exercises,
- swing exercises, and
- ballistic exercises.

Functional training = Action + Function

Let's never forget it.

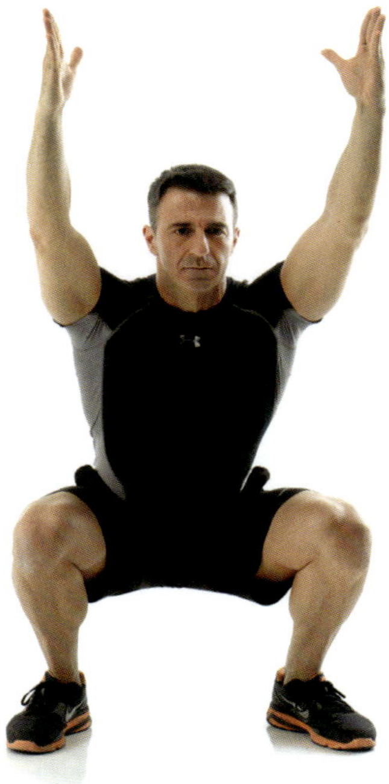

1 Bosco C. and Viru A. (1996) *Biologia dell'allenamento*, SSS, Roma

6.2 ACTION AND FUNCTION OF THE LOWER BODY

The function of the coxofemoral joint and of the muscles which originate or are inserted nearby confirm the necessity for functional training of the lower body.

The muscles in the joints of the lower body contrast the effect of gravity and of any other force that tends to destabilize the body's balance.

The functions of the lower-body muscles are:

- Double support in the upright stance.
- Oscillation and support during locomotion.
- Transfer of the body from a lying down to an upright position.
- Sensitive information from the support points.

During ambulation, when one leg is lifted, the hip muscles are active in shifting the body weight onto the support limb and preventing the pelvis from falling down the side which isn't supported.

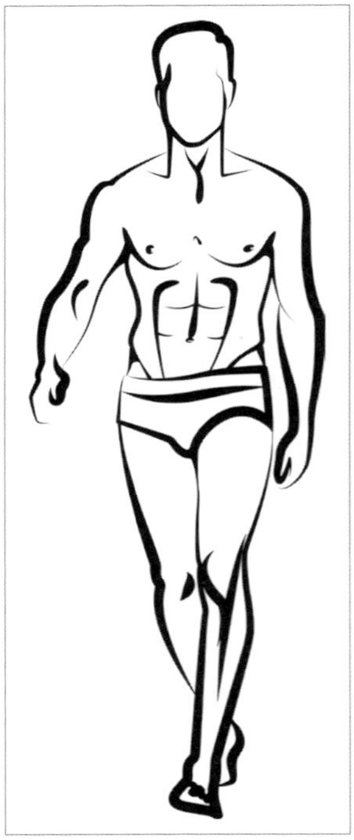

ADDUCTORS

They contract to shift the pelvis toward the support side; furthermore, they can act as hip extensors or flexors when walking or running, according to whether they are forward or behind the rotation axis. Finally, they stabilize the pelvis.

ABDUCTORS

When walking and running, they stabilize the pelvis on the support side, preventing it from falling.

ILIOPSOAS

It rotates the pelvis forward and is active in walking, climbing stairs, running or walking uphill, and getting up from a supine position.

QUADRICEPS

When running, it helps the gluteus to realize its maximal potential in the final extension phase.

GLUTEUS MAXIMUS

It is the body's most powerful muscle, the largest (66 cm2 [25.9 in2] in section) and the strongest. Its main action is the extension of the thigh on the pelvis. Its function is propulsion. This muscle is indispensable when running, jumping, and marching uphill.

FEMORAL BICEPS, SEMITENDINOSUS, AND SEMIMEMBRANOSUS

The femoral muscle group had already been reevaluated by the athletic training schools in Eastern European countries, and these evaluations are shared by American athletics coaches. It is a group of biarticular muscles (except for the short end of the femoral biceps), that ride the knee joint distally and the coxofemoral joint proximately. As such, their main action is the extension of the thigh on the pelvis, in synergy with the gluteus maximus, to which they also offer a great functional support in propulsion.

PIRIFORMIS MUSCLE

It is a hip abductor. Its action is maximized at a 60-degree flexion of the hip. It has an external rotation action before reaching 60degrees of flexion and an internal rotation one beyond 60 degrees. Pivoting on the femur, the piriformis inclines the pelvis contralaterally and tilts it backward. The piriformis is important because of its close contact with the sciatic nerve. Symptoms such as sciatic pains similar to those found in cases of herniated discs are frequent and attributed to an excessive shortening of this small muscle; curiously, they are also called "wallet-in-the-back-pocket syndrome", since the habit of wearing such objects seems to lead to articular compression and the shortening of the piriformis.

From this we can deduce that the main action of the coxofemoral joint and therefore of the whole hip extensor chain is propulsion. In order for the training of this kinematic chain to be complete, then, following the action-function principle, we have to add to basic and multijoint exercises of proven effectiveness (e.g., squats and lunges) and other exercises in which this function is expressed.

6.3 ARTICULAR REALITY: LONG-LIMBED AND SHORT-LIMBED SUBJECTS

We said at the beginning that articular reality, which varies from individual to individual, is an expression of functionality and therefore of evolutionary choices.

Among articular systems, the coxofemoral is the one that most exemplifies this evolution. Anthropologists have in fact noted how the shape of the femur—diaphysis, neck, and head—responds exactly to these evolutionary criteria. Its shape is variable and depends on functional adjustments. We can therefore distinguish two different types: the long-limbed subject and the short-limbed subject (Bellugue, P., 1963).

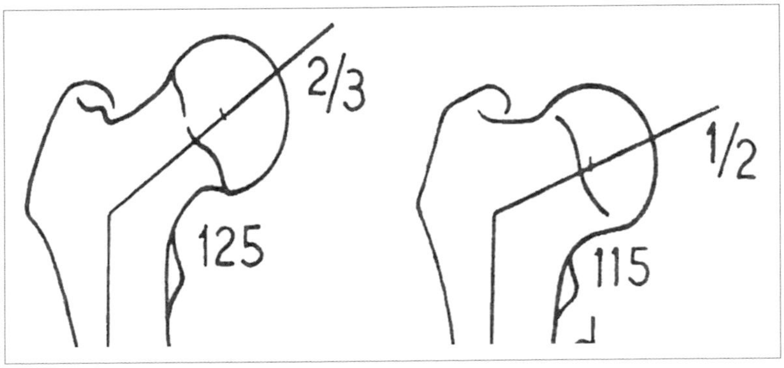

Femur head in long-limbed and short-limbed subjects (picture from Kapandji).

LONG-LIMBED TYPE

The femur head is a sphere 4-5 cm [1.5-1.8 in] in diameter for more than two thirds of the femur, supported by the femur neck which binds it to the diaphysis.

The femur neck axis forms with its diaphysial axis a tilt angle of 125 degrees and a declination angle of 25 degrees with the frontal plane.

The femoral diaphysis is thin, and the pelvis is small and high. This combination means a wide articular excursion of the femur head within the articular cavity, and this ensures great articular width, which can mean a talent for running. This subject is therefore suited to this type of activity (think of the Kenyan marathon runners).

SHORT-LIMBED TYPE

The femur head is barely larger than a half of a sphere; the tilt angle of the femur neck corresponds to 115 degrees, while the declination angle is about 10 degrees. The femoral diaphysis is short and thick. This combination means a limited amount of femur head excursion within its articular cavity. It is a morphology of strength. What the subject loses in terms of speed, he or she regains in strength and power.

6.3.1 Consequences

A specific anthropometric trait corresponds to a characteristic biotype.

Without dwelling too much on this, when we talk about biotype (from the Greek *bios* and *tupos*, meaning life print), we mean a group of individuals with similar physical, hormonal, personality, and other features. **The long-limbed type,** also called ectomorphs, is only slightly hypertrophic in both upper and lower body. It is an adrenaline-sensitive subject, with high levels of catecholamines and thyroid hormones and low levels of testosterone and androgens. It is poorly suited for weight training and tires easily and quickly.

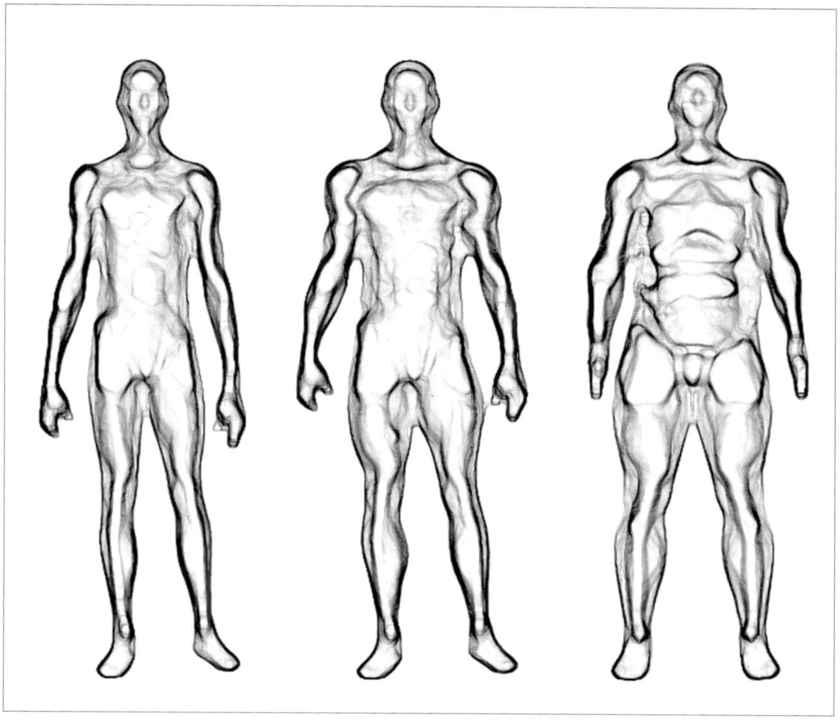

Ectomorphic, mesomorphic, endomorphic.

Training for this subject will need to be exclusively focused on long kinematic chains, involving large muscular areas; the training ought to incorporate the classic basic exercises and functional movements that are expressions of strength and power (skips, vertical and plyometric jumps, one-legged jumps). This is because we need to induce a strong hormonal response, especially at the androgen level, through training.

The short-limbed type, endomorph, has a greater propensity to upper- and lower-body hypertrophy. Generally, it has a low metabolism, great muscular mass and strength but also a propensity to gain weight. The female subject will have to pace herself in the basic exercises and include functional movements with aspects of endurance (uphill walking or walking) that do not involve white fibers. The male subject will easily increase muscular mass and will have to concentrate on slimming. A typical training program could feature one day of total body weights, one or two of circuit training, and possibly one day exclusively dedicated to aerobic work.

6.4 BACK ACHE, THE ILIOPSOAS, AND EVOLUTION

Evolutionary choices form the basis of functional training and explain the adaptations and changes our body has gone throughin the course of millennia. What we are today is the result of those choices. What is amusing is that we never think of ourselves as an outcome. So to speak, 6.5 million years ago we were a bunch of Australopithecines. The achievement of the upright posture is supposed to date back to about 2.5 million years ago. It represented a huge leap along the evolutionary scale. To explain this better: The life of an anthropomorphic monkey takes place over 10 square miles, while our hominid ancestor could cover this distance in just one day when hunting for food. Then followed the reversal of mandibular prognathism.

Coming to the present age, it is clear that evolutionary choices have always had biological and physiological justifications (we are, after all, the dominant species on the planet). We must proceed from here and think about the current issues. The most common pathologies in bone and joint muscular terms are back pains, especially at the sacral-lumbar level. The vertebrae that are statistically most affected are L5-S1 and L4-L5. At the heart of these aches there is almost always an excessive retraction of the hip flexors. The shortening of the iliopsoas—and even more common in sporting subjects, of the rectus femoris—is responsible for a more or less pronounced hyperlordosis; this attitude is favored by hypotonia of the rectus abdominis. The number one cause of these retractions is a sedentary life. Look at small children, and you will notice that they execute perfect squats with complete ease, and they easily hold a full crouch. Similar adaptations are still to be found today in several people on various continents. We have forgotten that man has evolved as a biped and as such must functionally discharge tensions and loads to the ground through a system of joints and shock absorbers: the joint capsules. The problem is that today, so statistics say, we stand up for only two hours a day and for the rest of the time we sit down on chairs, stools, seats, and sofas. A sedentary lifestyle doesn't fit with the evolutionary processes, albeit only progressively in older subjects. In all of these non-physiological positions, the support point for the locomotor apparatus is the pelvis in the sacral area. This is where we discharge forces and tensions for eight, ten, and even more hours every day, causing neuromuscular retractions as well. We could then ask why our body has chosen to preserve the iliopsoas despite all the problems it causes. We know that it is an important muscle for walking and running, according to Delmas' spinal index, but this feature has become more pronounced after coming down from the trees.

What about before? Why was it already there before? What is the function of the iliopsoas? We can use the following example to find the answer. A young man in a gym is performing chin-ups. For the first few repetitions, it all goes well; the body is perpendicular to the ground, and the execution is correct. Then fatigue sets in. What does our subject do? He bends the thighs into the pelvis. Why? Because in doing so he shortens the lever's arm and manages to complete a few more repetitions. Monkeys, from which we descended, execute the same movement when they move from one branch to another: They stretch and extend in the aerial phase, and shorten themselves by flexing their thighs and trunk during the traction phase. Also, when chimpanzees walk, they lean forward with their trunks and diminish the lordosis of their lower backs. Remember that the psoas muscle creates lordosis in the back by arching it. Monkeys keep using the iliopsoas, but they start from a lengthening position. Probably humankind has not yet adapted to the upright posture, and this would explain the dichotomy between the psoas function on the one hand and the use we make of it on the other. In general, seeing the difference between their action-function and current use, I believe it is always best to train these muscles by stretching them.

CHAPTER 7

7.1 PRESENTATION

When we talk about the abdominal fascia, we are discussing the most important area for the health of the bone-joint apparatus. The relevance of this whole area has come increasingly more important so that you frequently hear about core training. The abdominal segment connects the trunk and the lower limbs. The lumbar-pelvic region consists of:

- 35 bilateral muscles inserted in the pelvis.
- 14 muscles that link the pelvis to the spine.
- 21 muscles that connect the pelvis to the lower extremities.

The abdominal corset (picture from Kapandji[1]).

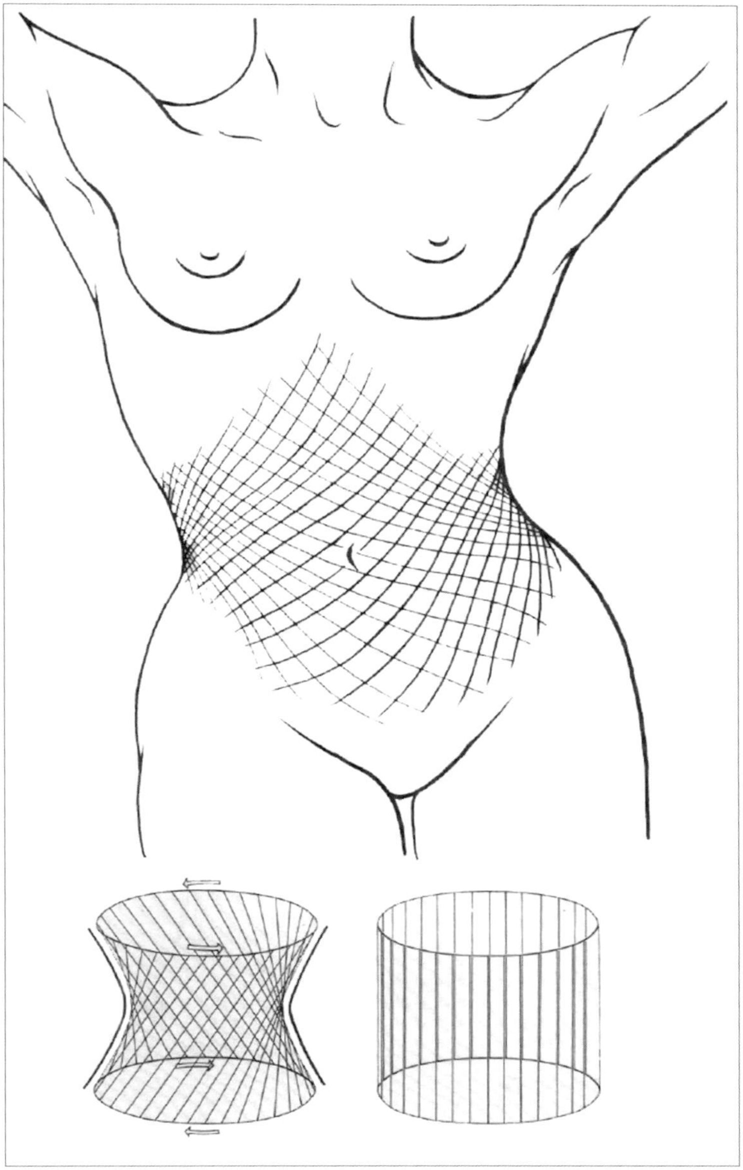

In the course of evolution, the rachis has changed from being a link between upper, anterior limbs and lower, posterior limbs to an antigravity support structure with static and dynamic features. In the presence of hypotonia of the rachis musculature, we assume incorrect and deficient postures which may lead to spine problems, such as postural defects, or pathologies, such as hyperlordosis, hyperkyfosis, or worse, scoliosis. A strong athlete will have a strong abdomen and toned, efficient abdominal fascia.

1 Kapandji I.A (1983). *The Physiology of the Joints*, Elsevier Churchill Livingstone Publisher.

7.2 CORE

The functions of the abdominal fascia are stabilization, motion, and control. But we are specifically talking about these muscles:

- Rectus abdominis
- Transversus abdominis.
- Internal oblique muscles.
- External oblique muscles.
- Quadratus lumborum.
- Erector spinae.
- Pelvic floor muscles.

We may think of the core as a bucket. The cylindrical supporting structure consists of three strata of muscles: the transversus abdominis and the oblique muscles. The anterior securing hinge is the rectus abdominis, and the posterior hinge is made of the erector spinae muscles and the quadratus lumborum. The bottom of the bucket is made by the pelvic floor muscles.

7.3 PELVIC FLOOR

The pelvic floor is a group of muscles which creates a weave among the pelvis bones. In the course of evolution, with the shift from a horizontal, quadrupedal or semi-quadrupedal posture to the upright posture, the pelvic floor muscles have decidedly changed their function. If before their almost exclusive function was waste expulsion and synergy in parturition, now with the bipedal posture they have acquired the role of support platform for the organs and the abdominal cavity. In the female subject, the poor activation of pelvic floor muscles is the cause of frequent pathologies, especially post-childbirth complications, from incontinence to the prolapse (a collapse) of the uterus.

7.4 ACTION OF THE ABDOMINAL FASCIA

The core's complexity relates primarily to its muscles.

RECTUS ABDOMINIS

This muscle flexes the trunk forward and laterally; it raises the pelvis and participates in abdominal pressure. It plays an important role in maintaining the correct posture of the pelvis, as an antagonist to the quadratus lumborum. It is a muscle with an important aesthetic value, but, functionally speaking, it is secondary to the large abdominal muscles.

EXTERNAL OBLIQUE MUSCLE

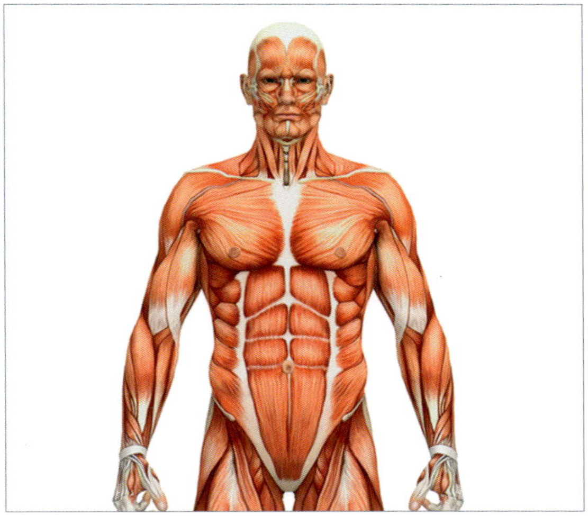

This muscle is synergistic to the rectus abdominis in the flexing of the trunk. It tilts the trunk laterally and turns it contralaterally (the right external oblique muscle turns the trunk to the left, and vice versa). It participates in the final rotation extension in all the throwing movements practiced in athletics such as rugby, tennis, baseball, golf, and even boxing. Every time we apply a weight to one side of the body (e.g., carrying a suitcase or a dumbbell), the oblique muscles on the opposite side contract in order to stabilize the trunk and prevent it from falling laterally. It is part of the abdominal corset.

INTERNAL OBLIQUE MUSCLE

This muscle shares in the forward flexion of the trunk; it tilts the trunk laterally or turns it toward the contracting side. In rotation, it is synergistic with the rectus abdominis and the external oblique muscle on the opposite side. It contributes to abdominal pressure.

TRANSVERSUS ABDOMINIS

This muscle's main activity is abdominal pressure: It holds back the viscera and stabilizes the pelvis. It is thanks to the synergy between the transversus abdominis and the oblique muscles that the pelvis and the lumbar tract acquire strength and stability.

QUADRATUS LUMBORUM

As the name itself suggests (*quadratus* means "square" in Latin), this is a square-shaped muscle that goes from the iliac crest to the spine and the ribs. It tilts the trunk backward and laterally. It is the real antagonist of the rectus abdominis.

ERECTOR SPINAE AND LATISSIMUS DORSI

Their action is the extension and lateral tilt of the back.

7.5 FUNCTION OF THE ABDOMINAL FASCIA

Let's start talking about the function of the abdominal fascia muscles beginning from the synergy between the diaphragmatic and the mediastinal cavities that border each other. They are physically divided but functionally associated. With inspiration, when the thorax expands, the mediastinal cavity is depressed; with expiration it is the diaphragmatic cavity which is depressed, while the mediastinal cavity expands. Endo-abdominal or peritoneal pressure increases during an effort, especially when it is combined with forced expiration (Zatsiorskij and Sazonov[2], 1988). As a result of the internal support, pressure on intervertebral discs may be reduced by 40%; it is produced by the activity of the abdominal wall, intercostal, and diaphragm muscles.

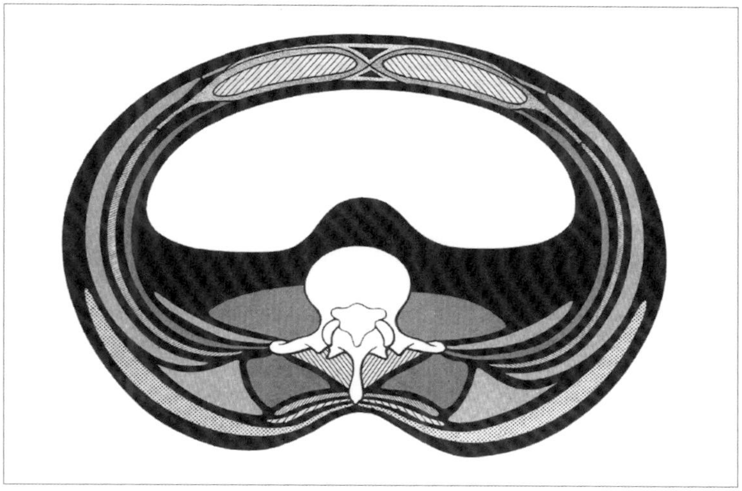

The pelvis (picture taken from Kapandji[3]).

The picture of the pelvis (from Kapandji) reproduces a cutaway of the mediastinal cavity from which the action of the large muscles of the abdomen is evident: the external oblique, the internal oblique, and the transversus abdominis. These three muscles warp the abdominal cavity in three superimposed circles, joining at the front in a fibrous aponeurosis, into the weave in which the rectus abdominis is inserted. This already shows us that it is almost useless to work on the rectus abdominis to reduce the waistline because it doesn't have much influence. For this purpose we ought instead to focus on the three previously mentioned muscles. The abdominal fascia function as:

2 Zatsiorskij V.M. and Sazonov V.P. (1988). "Basi biomeccaniche nella prevenzione dei danni alla colonna lombare durante esercizio fisico - Revisione della bibliografia esistente", in *Atleticastudi*, 5.

3 Kapandji I.A (1983). *The Physiology of the Joints*, Elsevier Churchill Livingstone Publisher.

- **Stabilizers.**

Their role in containing the viscera and as stabilizers is ensured by isometric contractions which set the pelvis in an anatomic position. Let's think about it: If the erect posture is, or ought to be, the one most frequently adopted, our abdomen's number one function cannot be that of flexing the trunk on the ground, as with crunches and similar exercises, but rather it is the stabilization and rotation of the pelvis, working against gravity (does anyone do these exercises in gyms?).

- **Motors.**

The dynamic function is guaranteed by anisometric contractions of those muscles which allow flexion, lateral flexion, and rotation of the trunk and lifting of the pelvis. Once again we are not talking about one single muscle but about a functional, synergistic set. The majority of these movements still takes place in the upright position. If we think about trunk rotation, we realize that the first and most frequent gesture of this type happens when walking.

- **Respiratory mechanisms.**

The abdominal fascia contribute to expiration and, in particular, to forced expiration. The latter is produced by the activity of the abdominal wall muscles, the intercostal muscles, and the diaphragm. In many sports where there are expressions of strength and power, it is a virtually physiological activation.

The visual and aesthetic effects of good abdominal corset firmness, and specifically firmness of the transversus abdominis, are several.

The firmer the transversus abdominis, the thinner the waistline is, since there is an accent on the curve which delimits it laterally and which coincides with the area between the ribs and the pelvis: the hip line (hyperboloid line). A firm abdominal corset implies a series of benefits, the most important being:

- Less stress on the lumbar rachis.
- Greater core strength owing to the action of the pivot muscles.
- Reduction of back pains, owing to the increased stabilizing function.
- Reduced visceral ptosis.
- Improved synergy between lower and upper limbs in the work of kinematic chains.

7.6 THE CENTRIFUGE PRINCIPLE

In training theory, the core's importance is confirmed by its first-place ranking in the sequence of muscular areas to be trained in beginners: the centrifuge principle. This because the abdominal fascia and the joints which rely on it are the fulcrum upon which the forces coming from the upper body and the stress coming from the lower limbs (impact with the ground) are discharged. It is not by chance that the rachis is the area most subject to wear and to inflammatory pathologies: back pains, sciatica, and lumbago. And it is no less by chance that the back pains of 50-year-olds are becoming a heritage of the younger generations.

CHAPTER 8

SCAPULOHUMERAL GIRDLE

8.1 PRESENTATION

Only functional training allows us to determine instances of contradictions in our locomotor apparatus.

The scapulohumeral joint is a case in point. It is an enarthrosis, like the coxofemoral joint. In other words, it has a greater range of movement compared to other joints.

Unlike the coxofemoral joint, however, where trunk weight contributes to the stabilization of the femur head within its articular cavity, in the scapulohumeral joint, the humerus is simply hanging from the trunk. In fact, when the deltoid muscle is at the point of maximum contraction with the arm abducted at 90 degrees, the humerus head deviates from the line of articular constraint.

The conformation of the shoulder joint tells us that our bodies' evolutionary choice has been one of mobility at the expense of stability.

The humerus head, in fact, only partially adheres to the glenoid cavity, remaining mostly outside the articular constraint.

Rather than entering the glenoid cavity, the humerus hangs from the trunk and moves in different directions. It is able to do this because of its active stability, created by the development of the nearby musculature, and its passive stability, ensured by the same muscles' tendons and by the ligaments.

Besides the scapula stabilizers, the only muscles with a prevailingly stabilizing function are those in the rotator cuff, a real articular reinforcement structure.

Question: Don't you find it strange that all the muscles richest in white fibers are inserted on the most unstable joint in the human body?

- Triceps long head: 67% of white fibers.
- Trapezius: 64% of white fibers.
- Latissimus dorsi and pectoralis muscle: 50-58% of white fibers.
- Deltoid (anterior, medial, posterior): 40% of white fibers, located chiefly in the anterior part.

Yet white fibers tell of high workloads, expressions of strength and power, and great tension. On a joint that is unstable? Almost as a confirmation of this, anyone who has trained the scapulohumeral girdle muscles intensely, though correctly and without overdoing it, has been virtually obliged to suffer through painful and inflammatory pain in this joint. Why such problems? Where do they stem from? Read the next paragraph, and you will find the answer.

8.2 ACTION OF THE SCAPULOHUMERAL GIRDLE

All the muscles involved in the movements of the shoulder region are distally inserted on the humerus, scapula, and clavicle. These three bone segments share everything.

TRAPEZIUS

The upper band plays an important role in all traction and lifting movements; it lifts the shoulder and rotates the scapula. The medial band retracts the shoulders, bringing them closer to the spine.

The lower band rotates the scapula and depresses the shoulder in synergy with the pectoralis minor muscle. Besides, when contracted unilaterally, the trapezius rotates the head laterally. We notice it when we have irritating neck problems, in which the contracture of the trapezius or the sternocleidomastoid heightens the pains associated with them.

DELTOID

This is a powerful abductor of the upper arm. It can raise the arm above the head. The clavicular bands lift the arm forward; the acromion bands lift it up laterally; and the scapular bands abduct the arm backward.

Besides, it has an active stabilizing role for the joint, which it covers like a cap.

It is activated in arm circumduction movements typical of swimming and boxing.

It works in synergy with the pectoralis major muscle in all pushing movements along different planes.

PECTORALIS MUSCLE

It works in synergy with the deltoid's clavicular bands in order to flex the shoulder at 90 degrees.

It adducts and intrarotates the shoulder, flexing the arm on the transverse plane.

With arms raised and fixed, it pulls the trunk upward (the climber's movement). In all suspension and support movements, it prevents the lowering of the trunk together with the latissimus dorsi. It is also active in the forward lifting of the arm from the outside back position (discus throw) and from the below back position (bowling). It cooperates in deep breathing. The synergy of the pectoralis with the triceps is extremely important in explosive, fast pushing movements (i.e., sweeping aside branches and twigs). The long head of the triceps is in fact statistically the muscle with the highest percentage of white fibers.

LATISSIMUS DORSI

It is dedicated to the extension, adduction, and internal rotation of the shoulder joint. In all suspension and support movements it contributes to the stabilization of the trunk. It forcefully lowers an elevated limb (e.g., in throwing or hitting movements). It also pulls the trunk toward the arms. As we can see, it performs many movements in synergy with the pectoralis, to which it is often and wrongly considered antagonist. (How can two muscles with the same distal insertion, both acting as intrarotators of the humerus, be antagonists?) When the hand is above the head, the latissimus dorsi pulls the arm down and backward against the resistance, as if we were lowering a portcullis. In a climbing action, the hand is placed above the head, and the latissimus dorsi works hard to pull the trunk toward the arms, lifting the whole body upward. In subjects with a functional lower-body functional deficit, if it is impossible to lift the body from a seated position by extending the lower legs, the hands can lean on the chair's armrests and push and lift the body up, exploiting the adduction action of the latissimus dorsi as it lifts the pelvis. When walking on crutches, the latissimus dorsi helps the hands bear the body's weight (see how monkeys walk).

SERRATUS ANTERIOR MUSCLE

Its action consists of pulling the scapula forward around the thorax (protraction). This movement increases the ability to stretch the upper limb forward, adding strength to the gesture of hitting with a fist or overcoming a resistance ahead (i.e., sweeping asides leaves and branches).

TRICEPS

This muscle has both biarticular and monoarticular features. Its long end, which is biarticular, acts as extensor of the forearm on the arm and as extensor of the arm on the trunk. It helps the pectoralis major and the deltoid in extensions and thrusts, and it helps the latissimus dorsi as it retracts and adducts the arm.

It is the antagonist of the biceps and the muscle responsible for the largest part of the arm's volume.

BRACHIAL BICEPS

This is another biarticular muscle. Can you then explain to me why I often see it trained with the elbows blocked alongside the trunk, with a monoarticular movement? The biceps' proximal segment is covered by the deltoid and the pectoralis major. The biceps is a flexor of the forearm and of the humerus; it is also a supinator of the forearm. When the elbow is extended, the biceps tenses to contrast the force of gravity. It also acts as a help to the latissimus dorsi in tractions.

8.3 FUNCTION OF THE SCAPULOHUMERAL GIRDLE

What is the function of the shoulder joints?

As we have seen, the scapulohumeral girdle is an extremely complex crossroad of muscles, tendons, articular systems, and a kinematic chain that is the victim of an apparent incongruity. Yet it is simple: The scapulohumeral girdle is a transducer of forces, a functional hub. Exactly like a rail hub, purpose of the shoulder joints is to transmit the forces coming from the lower body or the trunk to the upper body.

The scapulohumeral girdle's function suggests exercises and execution modes different from those used now and in the past. It tells us, for example, that there is a contraindication to training the deltoid with a load applied to the upper limb only (e.g., slow forward movement and slow barbells) without the help of the lower chains. It also tells us that we cannot ask for stability with excessive movement control and slow-motion executions from a joint that doesn't have this feature. It is better to train it with exercises in which the thrusting action starts from the lower body and, with their help, is then transmitted to the upper body via the scapulohumeral joint. Exercise examples include: push-press exercises with dumbbells or barbells and jerk, clean, and press exercises. Paradoxically, training requires much higher loads for a shorter timeframe. This is what this articular systems demands. Actually, if you think about it, any sporting activity featuring a transmission of forces from the lower to the upper part of the body, such as boxing, baseball, tennis, golf, weightlifting, or martial arts, follows this line. You will enjoy greater results in terms of strength and hypertrophy, and pains, inflammations, sub-acromion syndromes, and contrasting syndromes will decrease or even disappear.

8.4 GRIP TYPES

Grip is an issue which is seldom discussed in gyms. It is generally thought to be a factor of secondary importance. However, there comes a time in training when the subject starts adopting a personalized grip, often based on unorthodox suggestions (the most common is: "use this grip, you'll feel the pectoralis better"). Actually, strength stems from the grip. Power grips bring the maximum amount of the sensitive area of the fingers and the palm of the hand in contact with the object being gripped. The four fingers flex around the object while the thumb wraps around the opposite side; this way the sensitive receptors of the areas involved ensure there is the right pressure for controlling the barbell. In this action, all the muscles in the fingers and thumb that close the hand are active: the muscles of the thenar eminence and the hypothenar stabilize the palm's medial side against the object, the finger muscles grab, and the wrist extensors impart a stable base to the gripping action. Pay attention to when you close your fist; notice the hand, wrist, and forearm become one single functional block, a single segment. The harder the hand grips an object, the greater the wrist extensors' activity is and the more extensive the central nervous system's motor signal is. One of the primary reflexes in a newborn baby is flexing the fingers when pressure is exerted on the center of their palm. This kind of grip and the physiological reactions which subsequently intervene increases nerve response and muscular fibers recruitment.

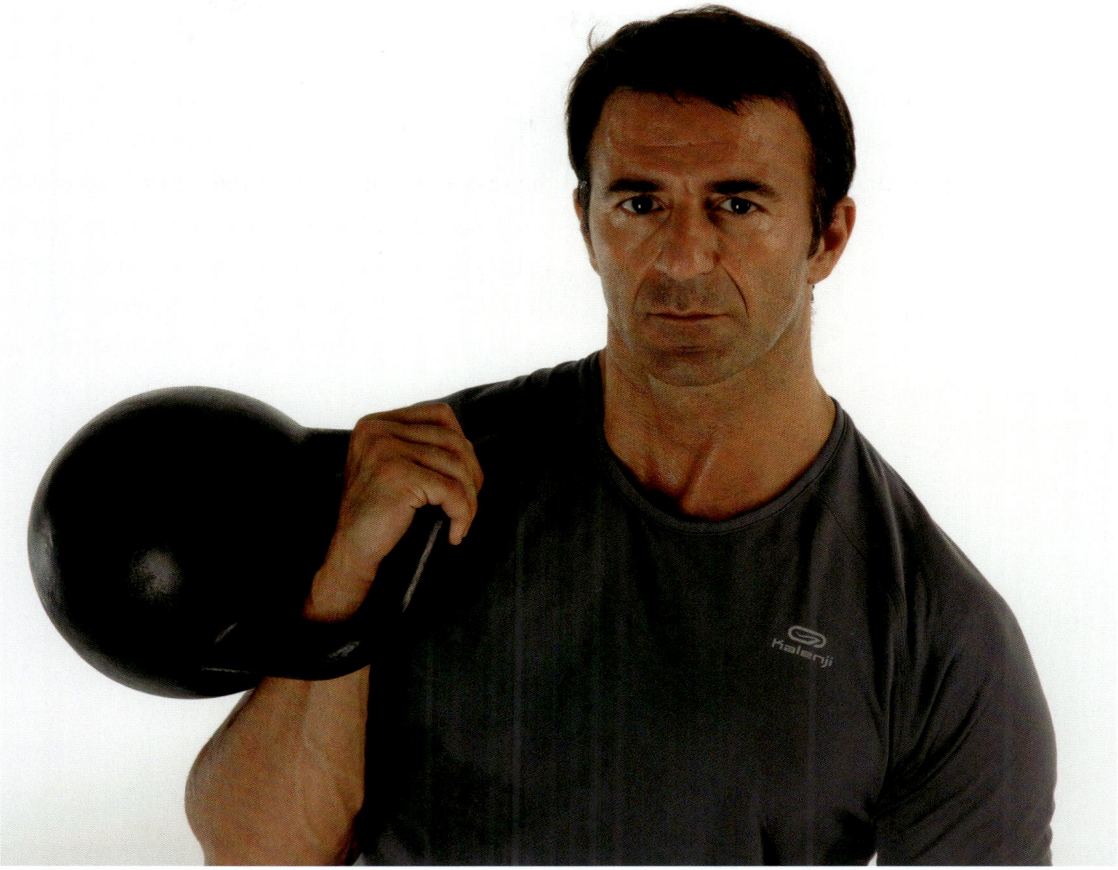

CHAPTER 9

9.1 PRESENTATION

The peculiarity of the foot is that it is the only part of the human body in continuous contact with the ground. While the vast majority of animals stand and ambulate on their fingers (digitigrade), man is a plantigrade (i.e., he or she rests the whole sole of the foot on the ground). When we stand, the ground exercises a force which is equal to and opposite to our body weight called ground reaction force. This and other forces are applied to the inferior limb joints—pelvis, knee, and ankles—which for this reason have a very high functional synergy. The role of the foot and ankle joints is:

- To orient the foot in order to set the sole correctly on the ground.
- To modify the shape and curvature of the plantar arch in order to adapt the foot to the ground's asperities and to create a system of shock absorbers between the ground and the leg.

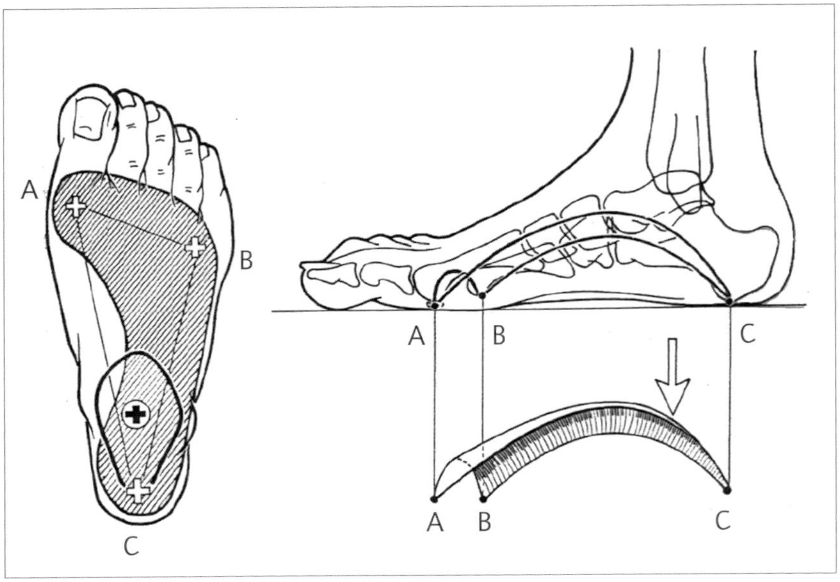

The foot (picture taken from Kapandji[1]).

9.2 WALKING

In terms of the tibial-tarsal joint, the posterior tibial, gastrocnemius, and soleus are the muscles chiefly responsible for propulsion when walking, running, and jumping. The action of the calf muscles is augmented by arching the foot and flexing the toes. When the heel leaves the ground, the toes extend, increasing the plantar arch. Walking is technically like a fall cushioned by the contralateral limb. In ambulation, we have a foot-plant phase for approximately 60% of the stride and an oscillation phase, with the foot off the ground, for about 40%. This means there is an alternation of monopedal support and bipedal support phases. At the start of the foot-plant phase, the foot is forward of the trunk and pushes ahead and toward the ground, decelerating the body's fall and providing support. In the final phase, though, the foot is at the rear of the body and pushes down and backward, providing acceleration. Let me underline the intervention of the upper body in ensuring a correct, coordinated posture as a confirmation of our physiological conformation based on kinematic chains.

1 Kapandji I.A (1983). *The Physiology of the Joints*, Elsevier Churchill Livingstone Publisher.

9.3 RUNNING

When running, the percentage ratios change drastically: the foot-plant phase ranges between 40 and 27%, depending on speed .The faster the athlete is, the shorter the ground foot-plant phase will be (sprinters reach about 22%).

Running efficiency is the result of the accumulation and release of potential energy within the elastic component of the tendons and of the energy-transfer action by the muscles that stretch across the lower joints. The kinematic chain activated by the running action sets off and involves initially both the gastrocnemius and the soleus. Both muscles help the action of the plantar arches and the forefoot. Then, in sequence, it involves the quadriceps, the hip extensor chain (femoral biceps and gluteus), and the abductors, compensating for the pelvis' fall at the foot plant. In terms of the foot, the action of the astragalus is essential. This is the bone that partitions the forces applied by the ankle and the tibia during the various phases. Because of the action of the plantar arches and the ligaments which run across the foot, the foot functions as a spring, ensuring the return of 80% of the elastic energy.

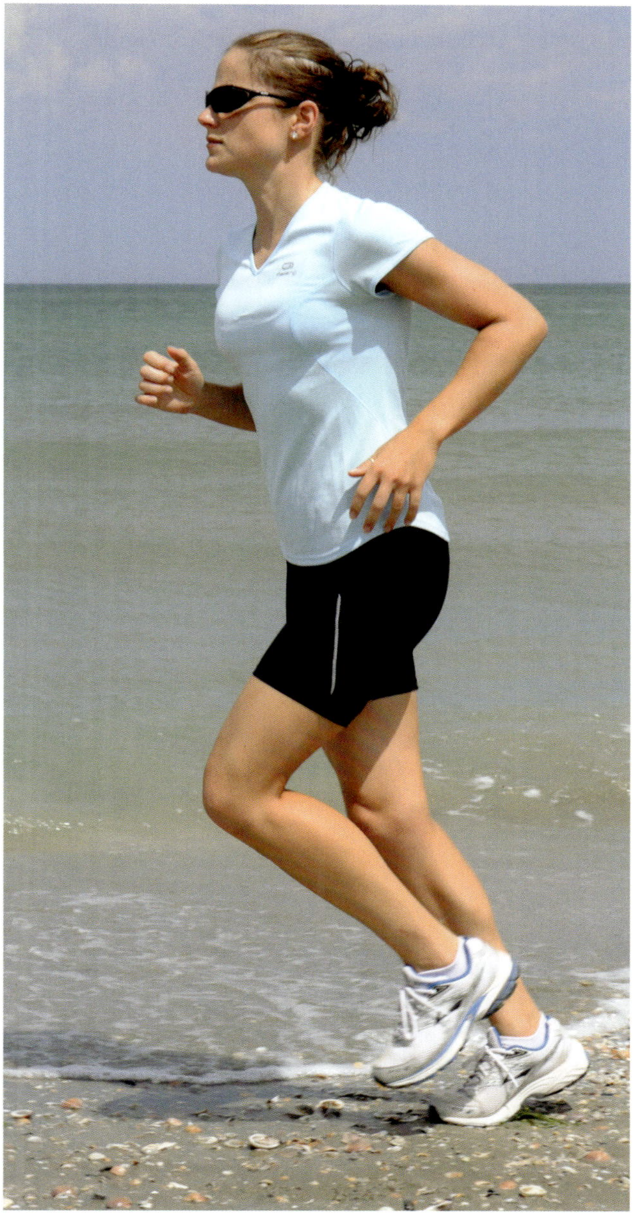

9.4 FOOT MOVEMENTS

As we have emphasized before, functional training points in one direction: training based on kinematic chains, following the evolutionary lines of the human race. It also suggests a different approach for gyms and sports centers: The action and function of a muscle, or a kinematic chain, should never be separated. We cannot disregard dynamic movements when training the musculature that runs across the tibial-tarsal joint, especially the triceps surae.

Let's think about it. These bone-joint structures have evolved for walking and running, and as such they have always been subjected to propulsive forces, both acceleration and deceleration. The exercises usually performed in gyms, even on machines, do not consider these features. It is a serious mistake to constrain our articular systems, which vary from individual to individual, by training only by the rectilinear path imposed by a machine. We have also seen how there is a synergy between the triceps surae and other muscles of the leg and thigh. It is obvious they have to be trained together in order to avoid a regression in terms of intra- and intermuscular coordination.

PART II – PRACTICE

CHAPTER 10

10.1 PRESENTATION

10.1.1 Origins

The medicine ball is one of the most ancient exercise tools for endurance and physical conditioning. About 3,000 years ago in Persia, sand-filled bladders were used by wrestlers for training purposes. In ancient Greece, Hippocrates used sand-filled animal hides for injury prevention and rehab. The modern medicine ball's origins date back to the end of the 19th and the early 20th century.

10.1.2 Types

The medicine ball is one of the most ancient exercise tools for endurance and physical conditioning. About 3,000 years ago in Persia, sand-filled bladders were used by wrestlers for training purposes. In ancient Greece, Hippocrates used sand-filled animal hides for injury prevention and rehab. The modern medicine ball's origins date back to the end of the 19th and the early 20th century.

The variety of medicine balls (shortened to med ball) available on the market is stunning.

We can distinguish among five types of medicine balls:

1. Rigid balls.
2. Soft balls.
3. Semi-rigid throwing balls.
4. Rope-bound or with handles.
5. Destabilized balls (with water or other material).

This classification doesn't exhaust the variety on the market but gives you an idea of the type of use that can be made of it and its differences. The exercises we will provide in this book refer to the first two types, as they are the most readily available.

10.1.3 Grip Types

Start by standing with feet shoulder-width apart and gripping the medicine ball in both hands. From this basic position, the type of grip can change with the exercise. Following are two other common positions when exercising with the medicine ball.

ZERCHER POSITION

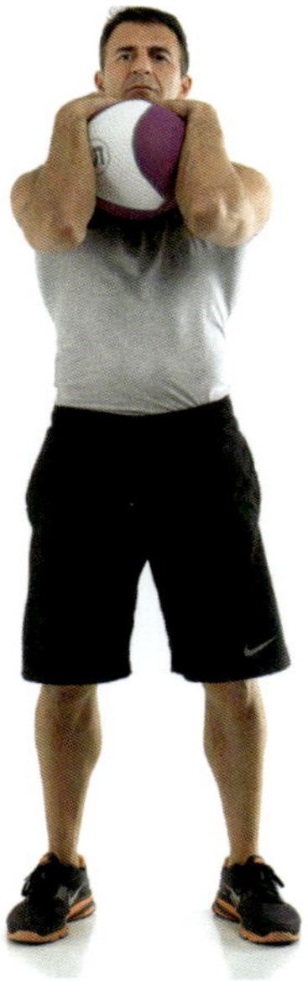

Execution

Visualize a soccer goalkeeper holding a ball tightly. The elbows are lifted out front in order to maintain the back's neutral position more easily.

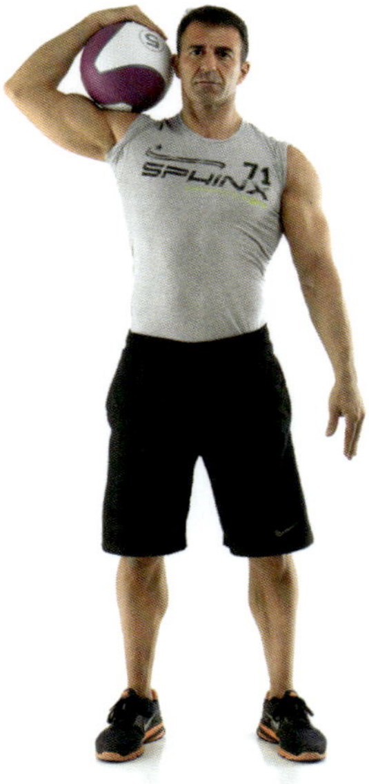

AT-THE-SHOULDER POSITION

Execution

Visualize a basketball player with the ball on top of the shoulder. The elbow is placed at an oblique angle to the body.

10.1.4 Exercises

An introduction is necessary. Any exercise can be completed using all four positions. Of course, to display them all every time would distract the reader's attention and also subtract space from other, equally important exercises. For this reason, when introducing an exercise in the following pages, I will present it in only one position, excepting for squats. You must be aware that the other positions are applicable, too, each with its own advantages. For example, in the at-the-shoulder position, we will have a greater stimulus, whatever the exercise, on the oblique muscles contralateral to the shoulder on which the medicine ball rests. In the Zercher position, on the other hand, we will have a greater activation of the paravertebral muscles. This type of work will be even more emphasized in overhead techniques, where force at the lumbar level is wanted and sought in order to prepare for heavy squats.

10.2 LOWER-BODY EXERCISES

MED BALL ZERCHER SQUAT

Starting position

- A | Adopt the Zercher standing position: med ball in your arms with elbows raised and pointing forward.

Execution

- B | Bend the legs with controlled movement and lower your body. Keep the arms raised, holding the med ball against your chest, throughout the whole movement. Keeping this position is an important part of the technique, because if you don't, you will tend to lower your elbows and the load will weigh forward, making the exercise similar to a classic squat.

A

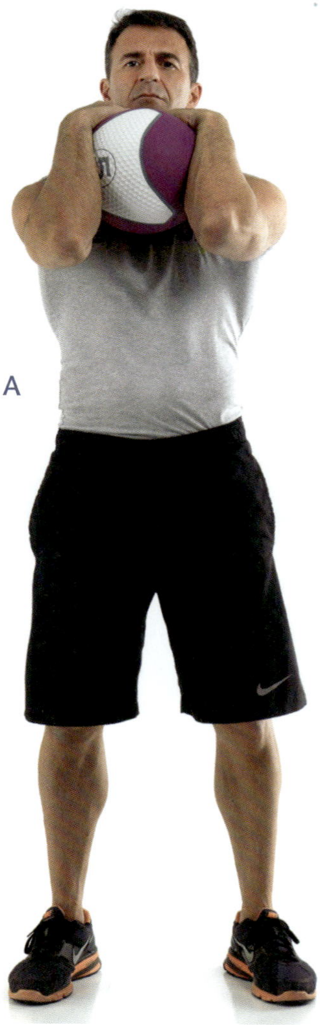

B

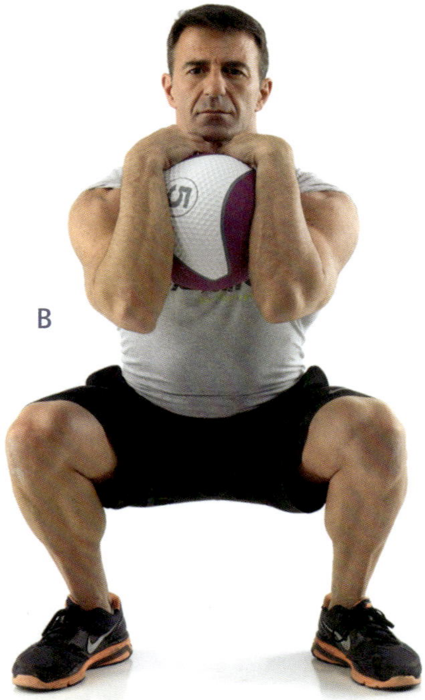

- C | Return to the standing position and repeat.

C

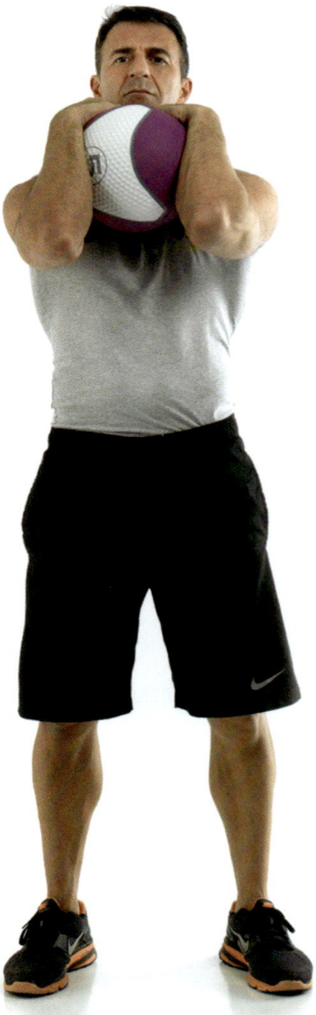

Discussion

This exercise is very similar to a frontal barbell squat, but it is performed with a lighter load, which makes it ideal for beginners or for subjects with specific problems. I regard it as essential training for barbell squats, which are heavier. I also consider it a preventive and even treatment exercise for back aches. Let's see its strong points:

- The movement is deeper than the classic squat, so it allows a greater and better activation of the gluteus maximus.
- It respects the load distribution on the spine's physiological curves better.
- It activates the whole paravertebral musculature in a balanced manner.

I will say no more: Get to work!

MED BALL ZERCHER SQUAT JUMP

Starting position

- **A |** Adopt the Zercher standing position: med ball in your arms, elbows raised and pointing forward.

Execution

- **B |** Bend the legs and sit back into a full squat with controlled movement.

A

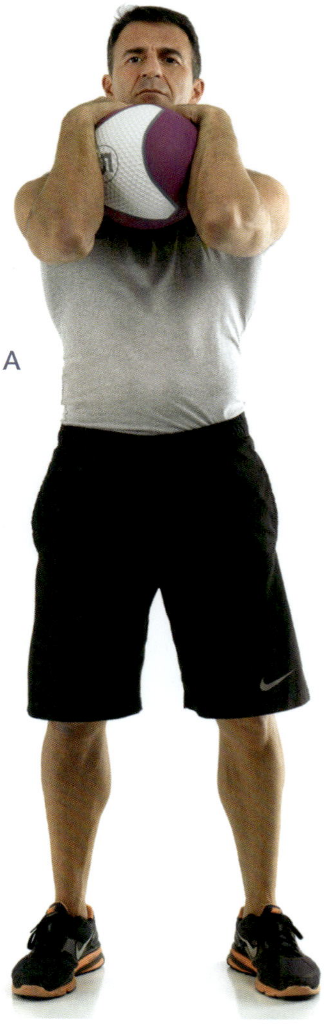

B

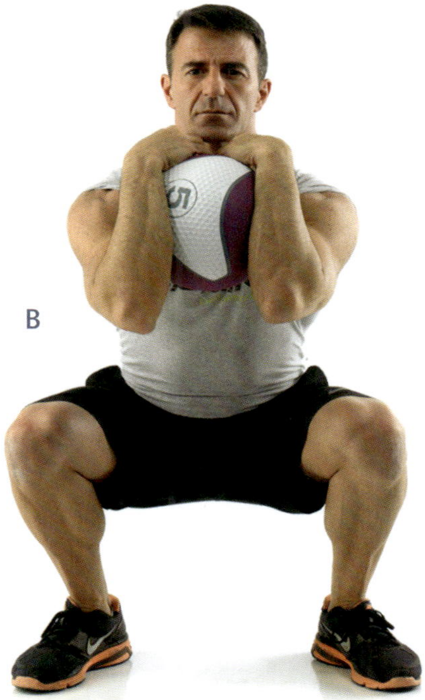

- C | Extend the lower limbs and jump up explosively. Land, recovering balance and stability, and then re-start, completing the required repetitions.

C

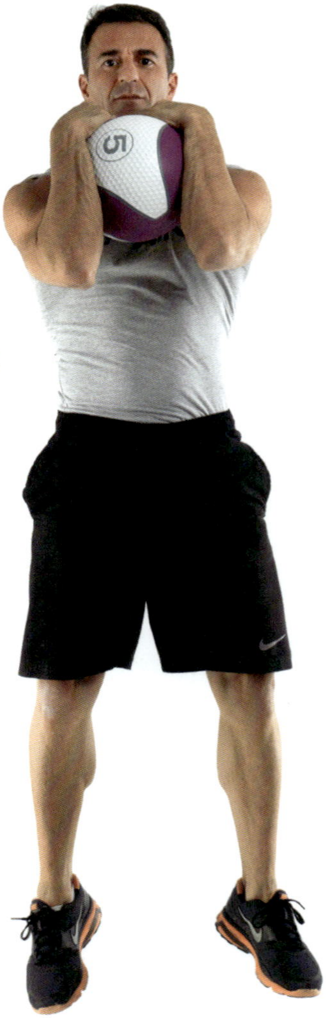

Discussion

The squat jump is an excellent functional exercise, so it is not by chance that it is included in all serious fitness programs. Compared with the barbell, the med ball is controlled and managed more easily. This version is an excellent way of teaching the exercise in order to transition from body weight to an overload workout. As in all ballistic exercises, the tendons, ligaments, and articular systems involved are under stress, which forces us to feature it in our programs with adequate timing and repetitions. Initially, I advise against more than 5 repetitions per set. It remains an exercise I will support entirely, as it combines action and function perfectly.

MED BALL OVERHEAD SQUAT

Starting position

- **A |** Stand with your legs at shoulder width. With straight arms, lift the med ball over your head in the overhead position.

Execution

- **B |** Bend the legs with controlled movement. Try to go as low down as possible, without modifying the spine's physiological curves. Stand up slowly and complete your set.

A

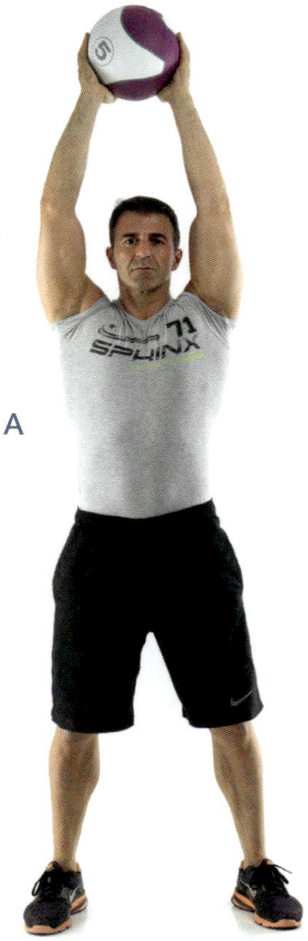

B

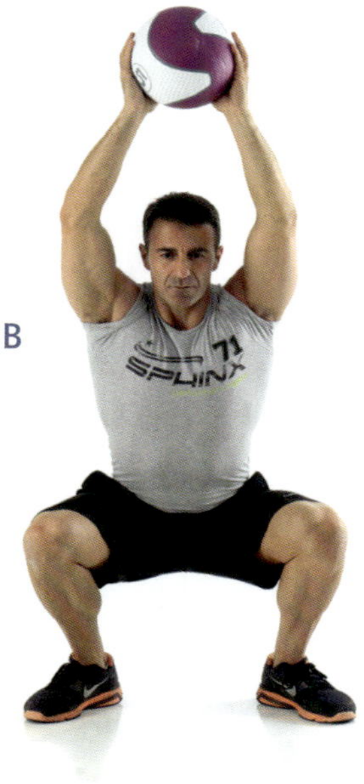

Discussion

I know, I've said it before, but repeating it is not hard: I adore overhead exercises! Pity this is a virtually unknown category in traditional gyms. These exercises yield much more in terms of results than what they require in terms of technique: activation of the parascapular musculature, in particular the humerus retractor muscles and the cuff stabilizers; and stabilizer work by the longissimus dorsi, erector spinae, multifidus, and the quadratus lumborum. Add the work on the lower body, and the picture is complete. In summary: posture and toning. Do you know many exercises with this kind of impact?

MED BALL JUMP

Starting position

- A | Adopt the Zercher standing position: med ball in your arms, elbows raised and pointing forward.

A

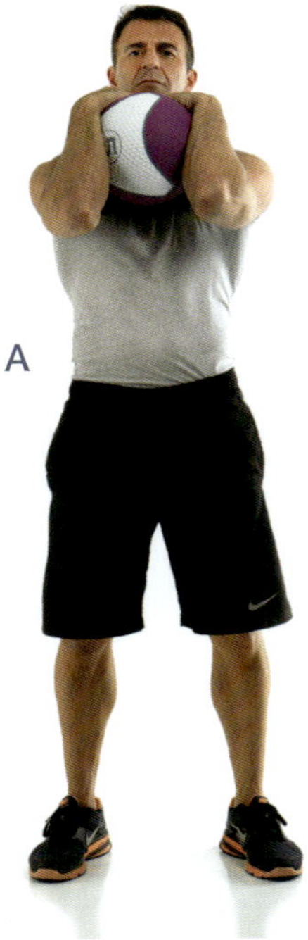

Execution

- B | Execute a brief, fast flexion of the thighs, and then jump upward.
  Land and stabilize.
  Start again.

B

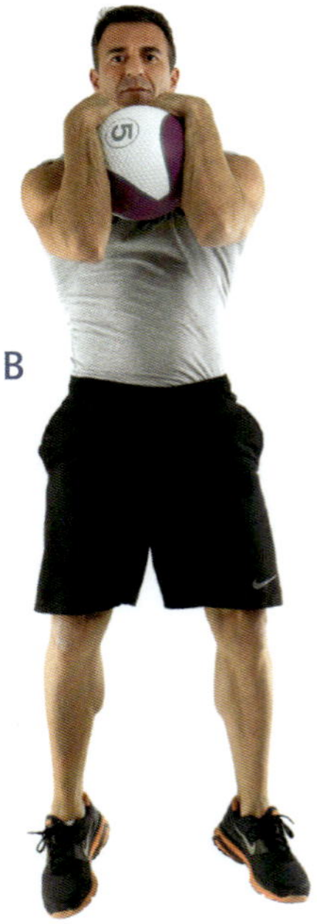

Discussion

We were born to run, walk, and jump. Thanks to sedentary life, a handful of years is enough to lose two of these skills. Only walking remains, but only if you allow for a pause between one shop window and the next. This should make us think. Do you realize how many people cannot jump anymore or are simply scared to do it? And how many coaches advise against jumps? I always repeat this: Sometimes the head coach inhibits the trainer, and the trainer inhibits his trainee. Feel free to return to your origins. Do it a little at a time, but do it. The hip extensor chain is activated by fast movements in which you can clearly recognize the function it was created for: propulsion. In how many gym movements do you find this feature? Practically none. The gluteus maximus, the femoral muscle, and the quadriceps are actively stimulated by this simple exercise. The abdominal fascia, quadratus lumborum, erector spinae, and the adductor muscles stabilize and absorb the movement thanks to the articular shock absorbers: the capsules.

MED BALL STEP JUMP

Starting position

- **A |** Adopt Zercher standing position; for greater ease, hold the med ball in your hands.
  Place one, two, or three steps in front of you, according to your fitness level.

Execution

- **B |** With a quick flexion-extension of the lower body...

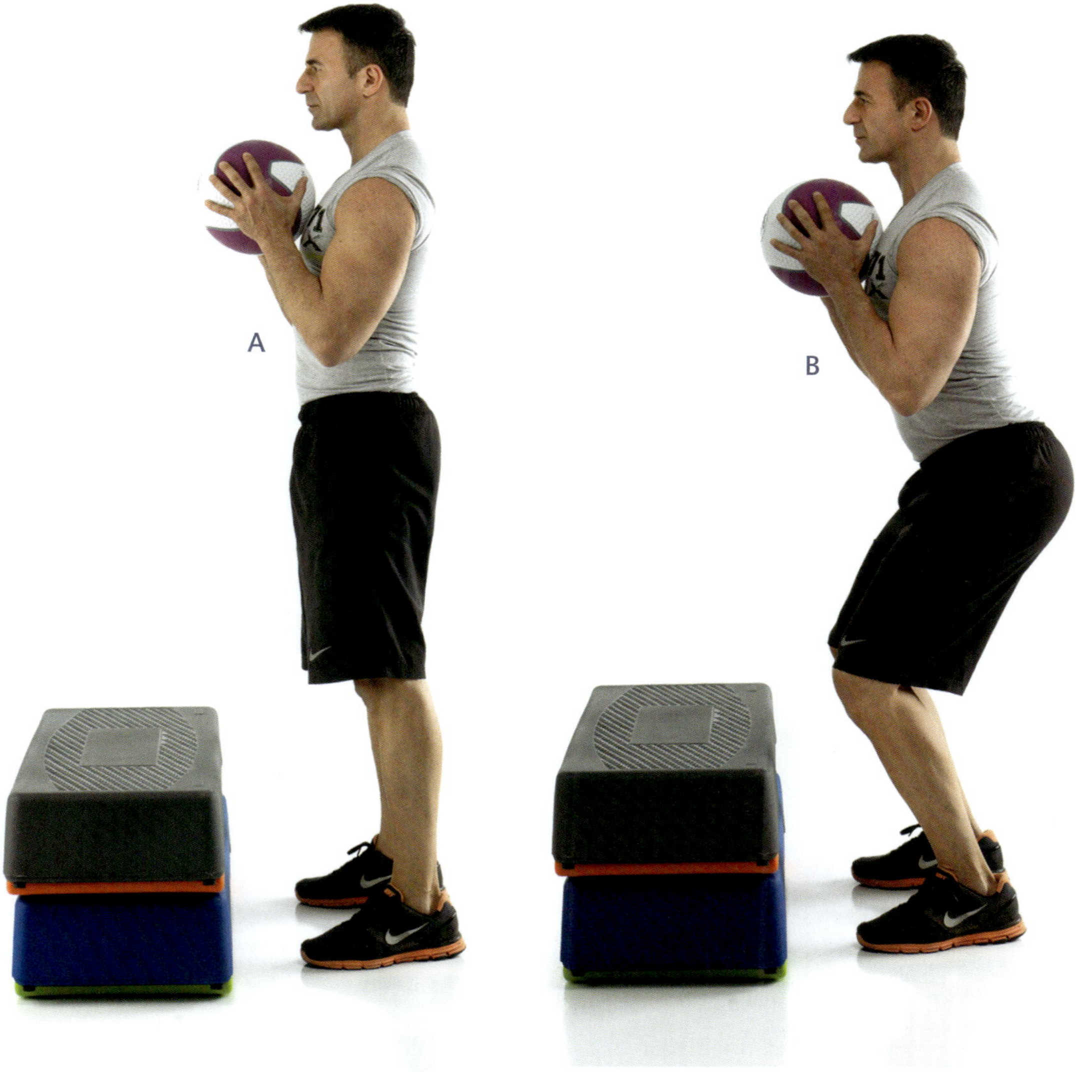

- **C |** ...take a short leap and jump on top of the steps. Take time to stabilize your position, and then return to the ground as if you were coming down from a high step (don't jump). Repeat for the required number of repetitions.

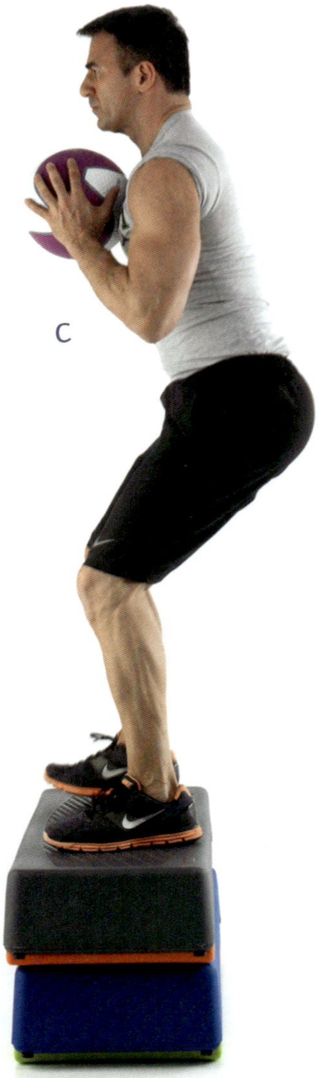

C

Discussion

The same that was said for the previous exercise applies here. The glutes, femoral muscles, and quadriceps are greatly activated in the propulsion phase; the abdominal fascia and the parascapular muscles work as stabilizers once you hit the ground. It is not a given that the level of difficulty here is greater. If, for example, the first instance was to jump on one single step (maybe even a low one), this may not necessarily be a more difficult objective than the previous exercise. How tall can a step be? 4 in. (10 cm), 8 in. (20 cm)? Yet you have no idea how scary it can be to execute a jump as small as this. Fear of falling down, of hurting yourself can make this exercise intimidating, though it is caused only by lack of practice in one of the movements that come more naturally to man: jumping. Set objectives: one step, two, then three, four, or even more, according to your fitness level.

ASYMMETRIC AT-THE-SHOULDER SQUAT

Starting position

- **A |** Stand and set the med ball in the at-the-shoulder position on top of your left shoulder.

  Set your right foot on a step, keeping the left foot on the ground; the legs are shoulder-width apart.

A

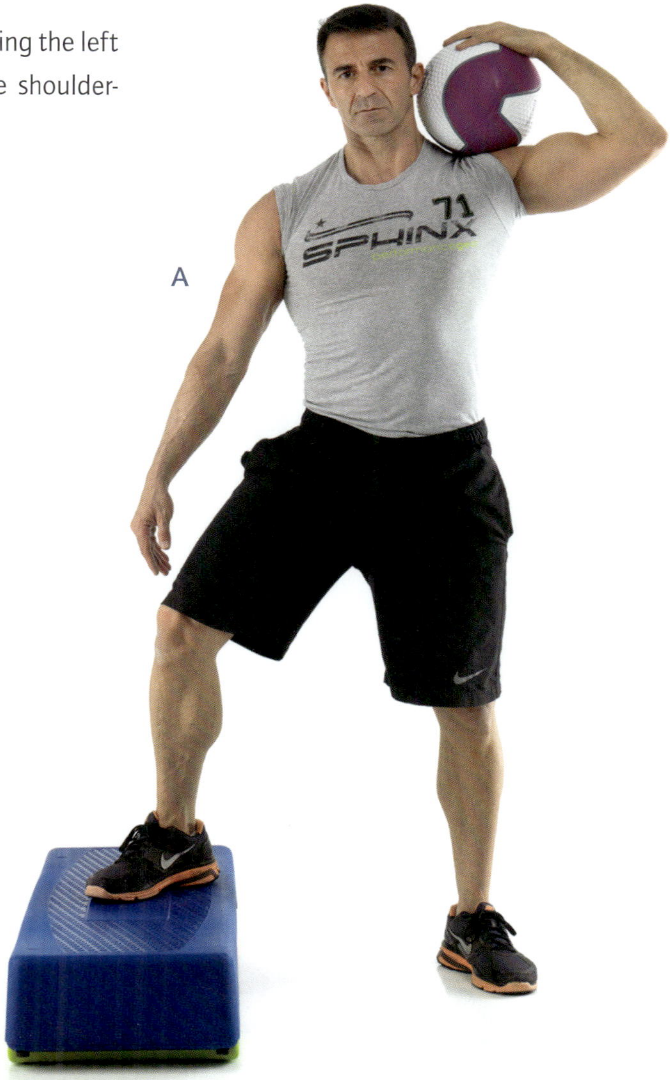

B

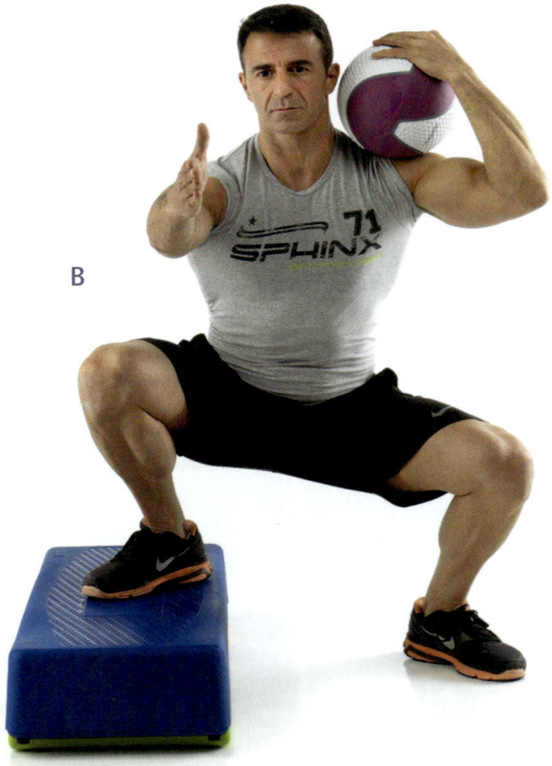

Execution

- **B |** With controlled movement, bend the legs and sit back into a full squat. Try to distribute the load on both legs and not to modify the spine's physiological curves.
  Rise slowly and complete the required repetitions.
  Change the legs' position (left foot on the step, right foot on the ground), and repeat on the other side.

Discussion

All asymmetric exercises reproduce situations found in daily life and in different sporting activities. Apart from cyclical sports and weightlifting, the body isn't perfectly balanced on both legs in any other activity. Asymmetric work teaches not only different, unconventional gestures but also a different type of recruitment and different intra- and intermuscular coordination. Furthermore, it stimulates articular mobility, especially in those joints (e.g., hip and the scapulohumeral girdle) which sedentary life tends to put in a plaster. This is a truly interesting exercise, but you will discover this only after trying it. Then you will really feel the kinematic chains working in a different way.

MED BALL SQUAT WITH ROTATION

Starting position

- A | Stand and hold the med ball in the Zercher position.

Execution

- B | With controlled movement, begin sitting back into a squat position. Then turn the torso to the right. As you descend, contract the abdominal fascia to protect the lower back and stabilize the torso.

A

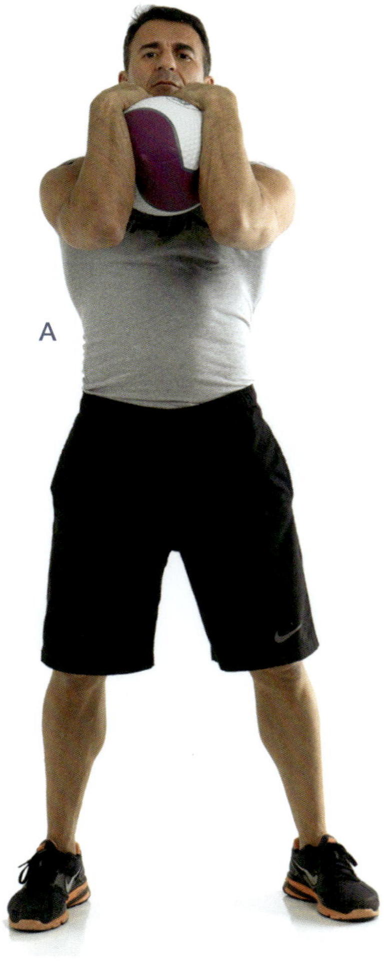

B

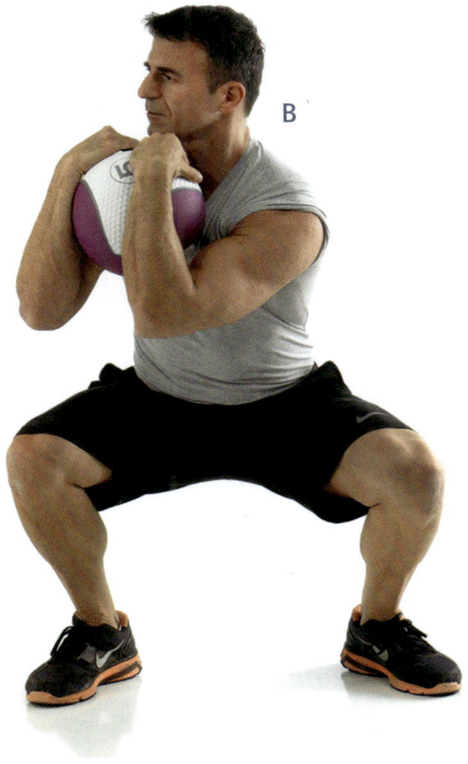

- **C |** Return to the Zercher position.

- **D |** Sit back into a squat, contract the abdomen, and turn to the left. Stand up again and complete the required repetitions.

C

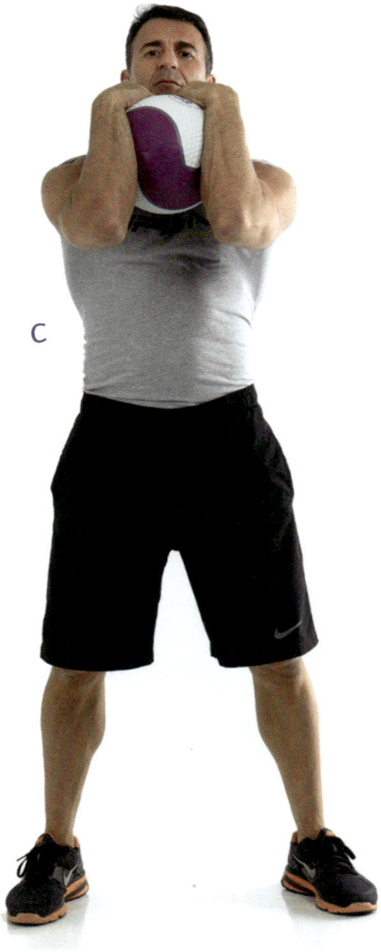

D

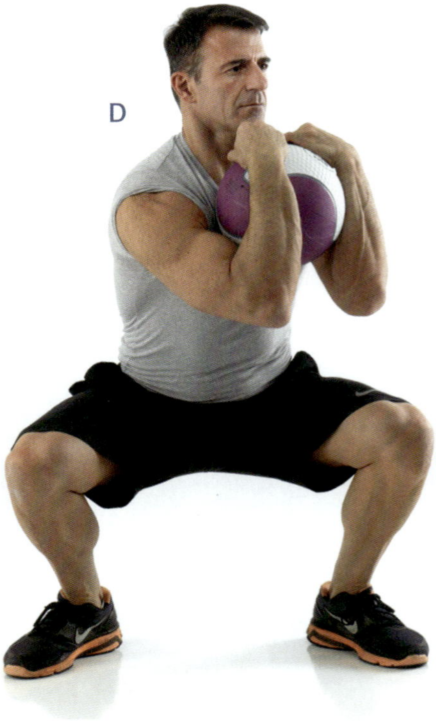

Discussion

This is a very simple, high-yield exercise. There isn't much to say about the squat; we are not discovering it today. What makes everything interesting is the torso rotation, which requires great motion control. During the rotation in the descending phase, it is essential not to modify the attitude of the pelvis and the legs (the natural movement would in fact be an intrarotation of the knee which is contralateral to the rotation's path). Contracting the rectus abdominis stabilizes the pelvis, limiting the range of torsion and protecting the lower back from excessive tensions.

MED BALL BURPEE

Starting position

- **A |** Adopt the frog position, with the hands resting on the med ball and the shoulders perpendicular to the hands to stop the ball from slipping forward. Distribute your body weight between the forefeet and the med ball.

Execution

- **B |** Leaning on the med ball, extend the pelvis and hips backward.

A

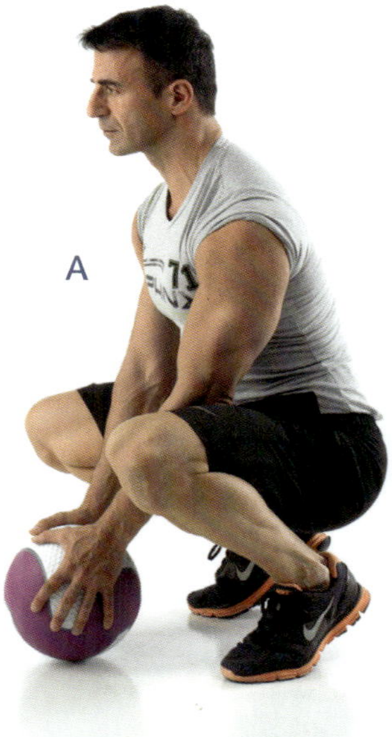

B

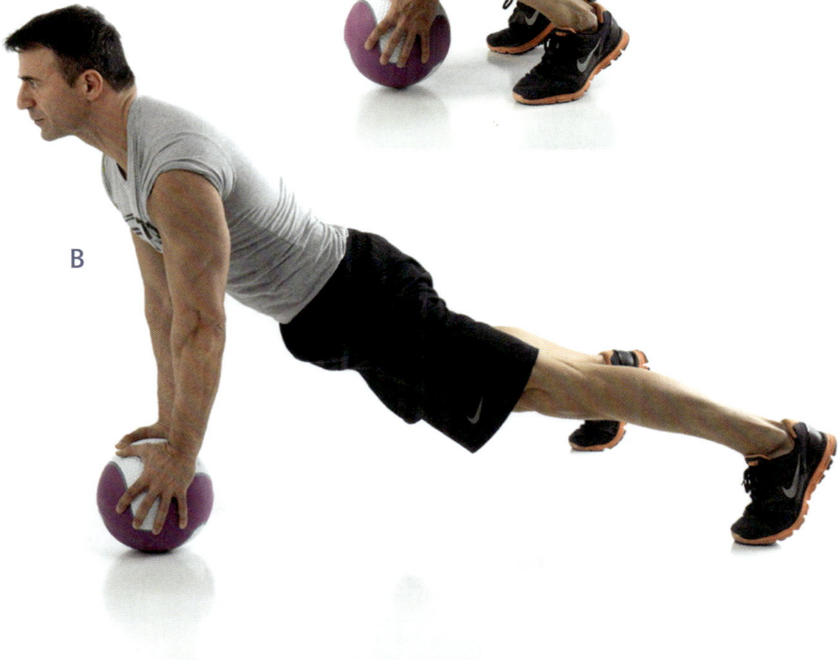

- C | Exploit the extension's elastic force to jump the legs back immediately to the starting position.
- D | Stand up.
- E | At the same time, press the med ball above your head. Start again.

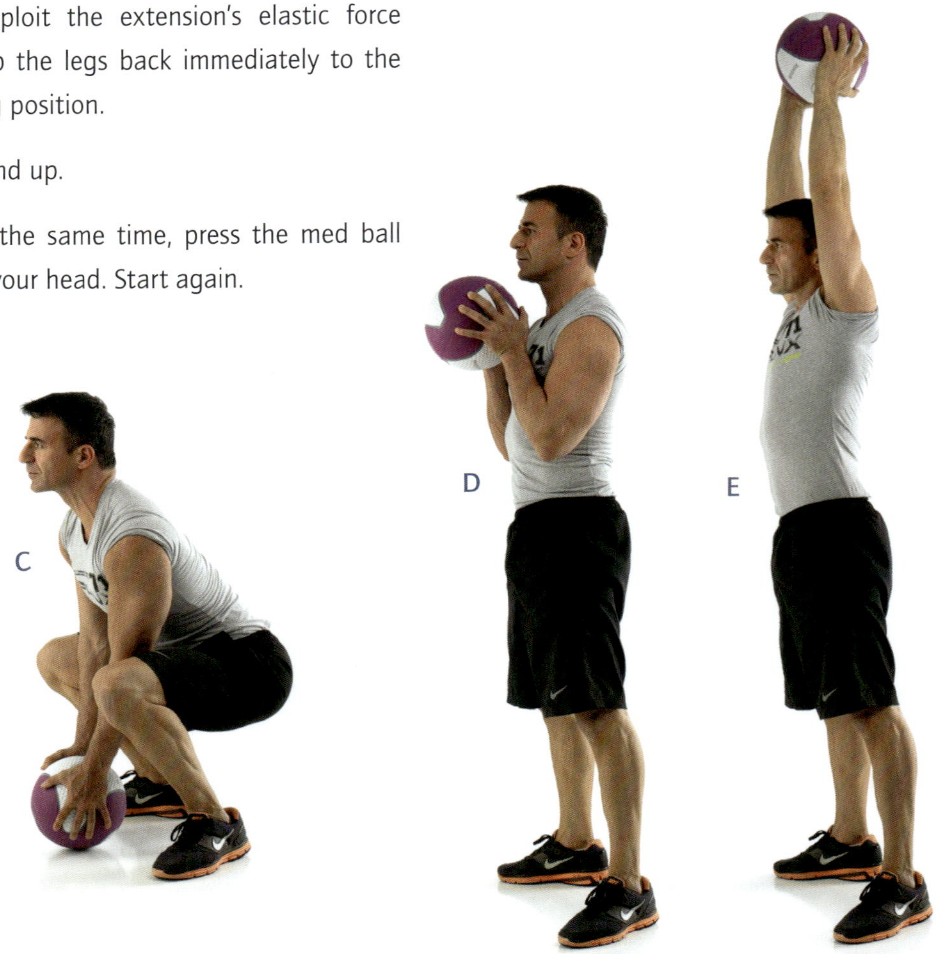

Discussion

The burpee is by itself a tough exercise which stimulates the whole hip and back extensor chain and the core as well. It is also excellent for articular mobility. Add the fact that in this specific execution the body's weight is on the lower body and the med ball (i.e., on a highly unstable surface), and you will already feel, even before doing it, how effective this exercise is. The following variations are also interesting:

1. For beginners: execute the burpee with the hands resting on the ground and only lift the med ball during the return phase from the squat to the standing position.
2. For intermediates: execute the exercise jumping up during the return phase from the squat to the standing position.
3. For advanced athletes: during the extension phase, execute a push-up with the hands on the med ball; in the return phase from the squat to the standing position, jump upward.

MED BALL DIAGONAL LUNGE

Starting position

- A | Stand and hold the med ball in the Zercher position.

Execution

- B | Bring the left leg forward and diagonally to the left (pivoting briefly on the right foot).
- C | Perform a lunge in place.

A

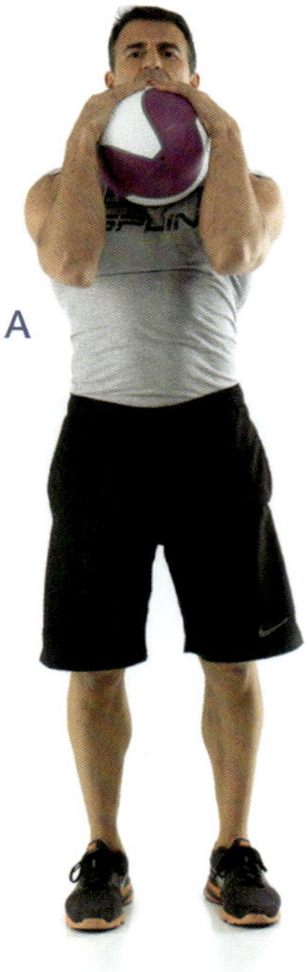

B

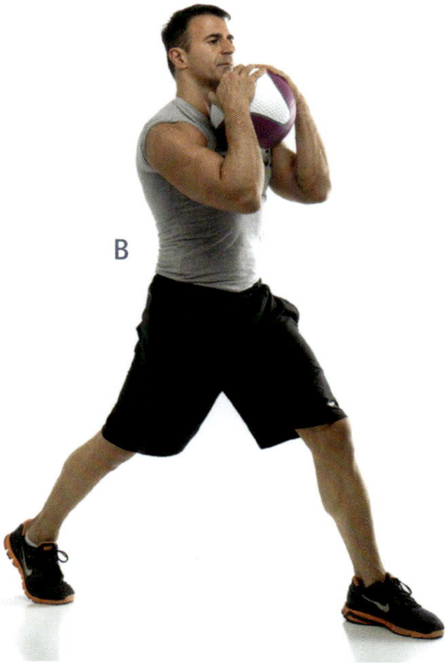

C

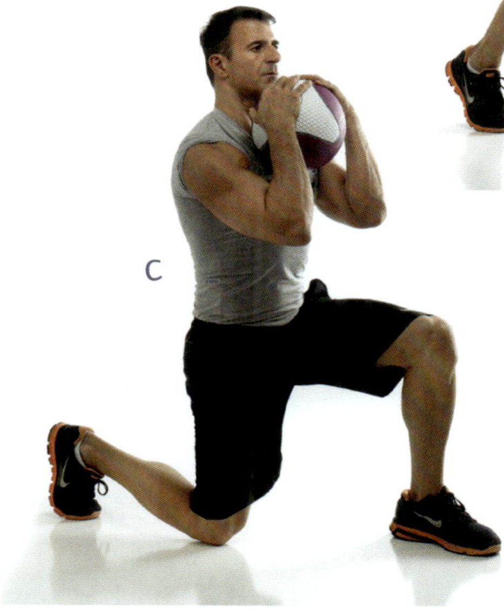

- **D |** Return to the starting position and bring the right leg forward and diagonally to the right (pivoting briefly on the left foot).
- **E |** Perform a lunge in place and then return to the starting position. Complete the required repetitions, always alternating steps in the two different directions.

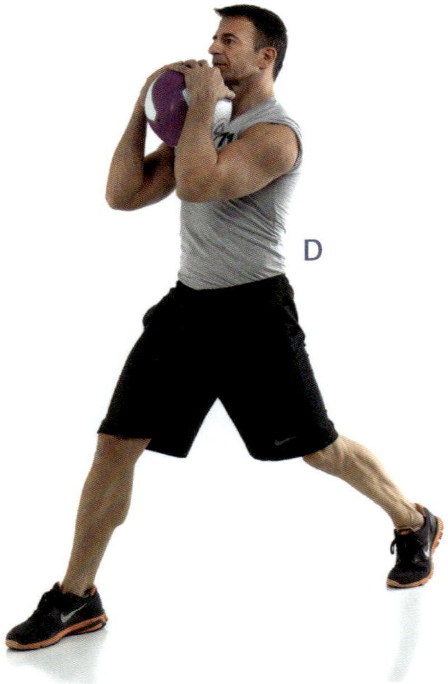

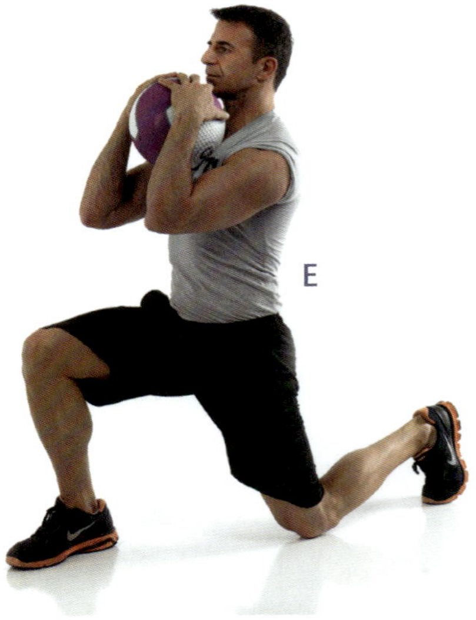

Discussion

The objective of this great exercise is to train the hip extensor chain, changing the movement angle repetition after repetition. Managing space in such a comprehensive fashion activates a series of nerve reflexes which influence balance, motor control, and proprioception. You also work on the abdominal fascia, which is subjected to contractions and extensions at alternate angles. An interesting progression on the same wavelength is to execute the forward and diagonal step to the right with the left leg and vice versa. Execution in this case will work more on balance and on the activation of the abdominal fascia. The progression of this exercise is the star lunge in which you have to work, repetition after repetition, on the entire 360-degree range. To give you an idea of the effects of this exercise, you need only to consider that it has been placed by Kibler at the top of the ranking in rehab protocols for subjects with injuries to the scapulohumeral joint. You have read right: This exercise was used to start the rehabilitation of people in a plaster cast or blocked on account of problems to the shoulder joint system. Because, let us not forget it, we are built with kinematic chains, and when you perform a lower-body exercise, something also happens in the trunk and upper body.

MED BALL WALKING LUNGE

Starting position

- A | Stand and hold the med ball in the Zercher position.

Execution

- B | Take a step forward with the left leg.
- C | Now perform a lunge.

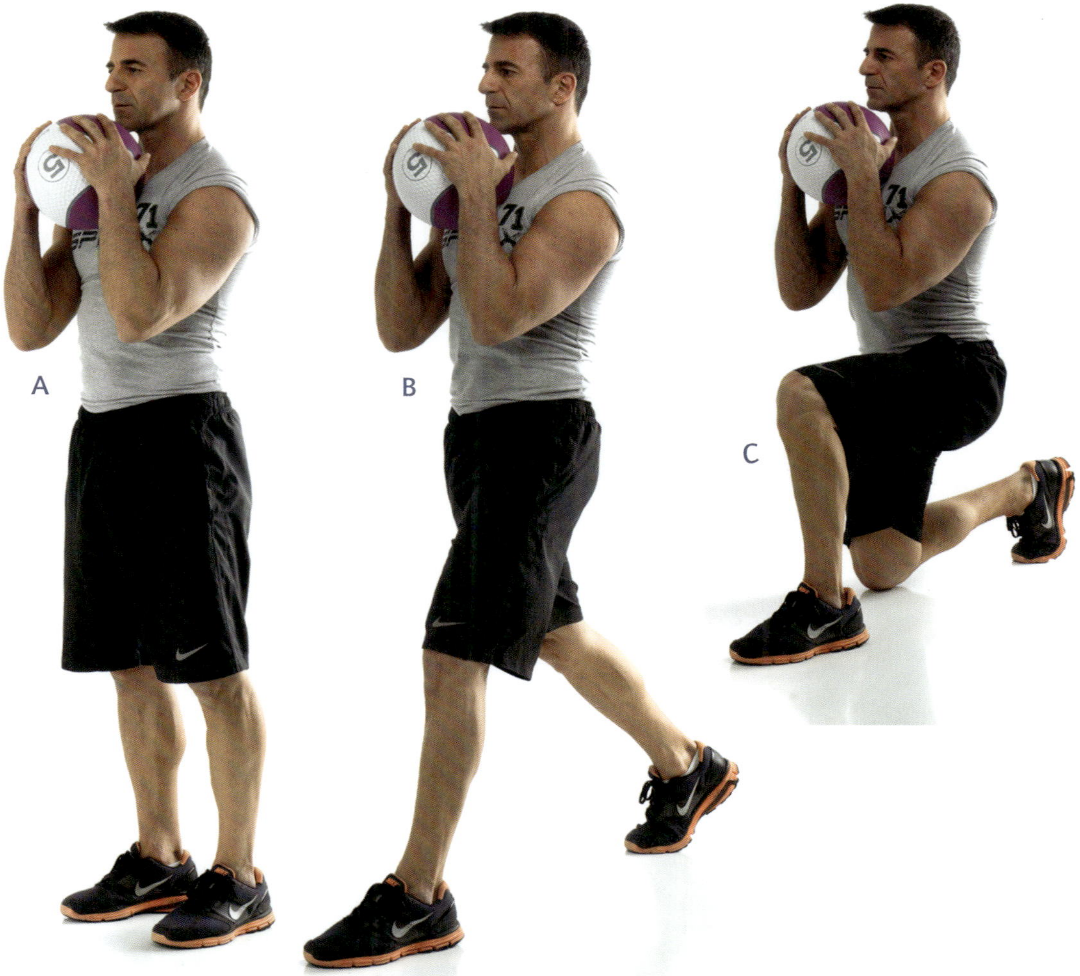

- **D |** From the lunge position, push the right leg up and step forward.
- **E |** Perform another lunge. Complete the required number of steps.

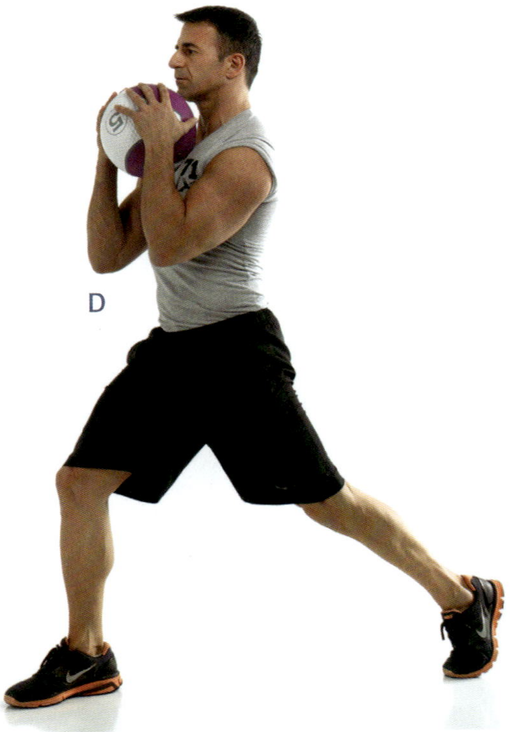

D

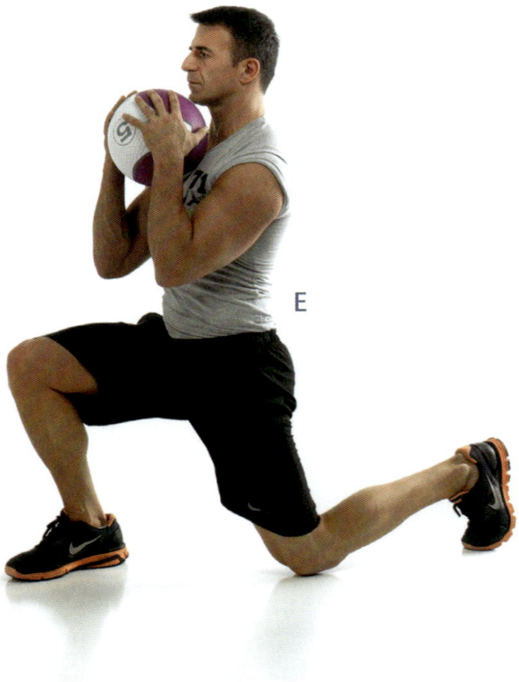

E

Discussion

The walking lunge is a functional exercise *par excellence*, one in which action and function combine perfectly. A very important element in its execution, explained in phase D, is propulsion. Many people believe they are doing this exercise when in reality theirs is a lunge in place, because from the lunge position they first lift themselves up and then they step forward. Read closely and execute to perfection. It is only when you are in the lunge position that you must push the leg up and forward: This is propulsion! Otherwise the thrust from the glutes will be equivalent to that of a simple stroll. In gyms, it is customary to execute in-place or alternate lunges, erroneously believing them to be the same thing. It is not so: Trying is believing. Circle this in red, and respect!

MED BALL SIDE-TO-SIDE LUNGE

Starting position

- **A |** Stand and hold the med ball to your chest.
  Take a step forward with the left leg.

Execution

- **B |** Perform a lunge, with the right knee brushing the ground.
- **C |** Rising up, pivot on both forefeet and shift from the sagittal to the frontal plane.

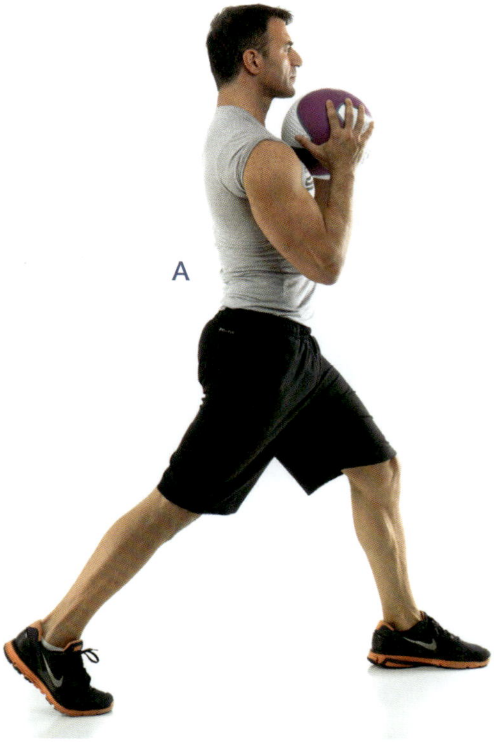

A

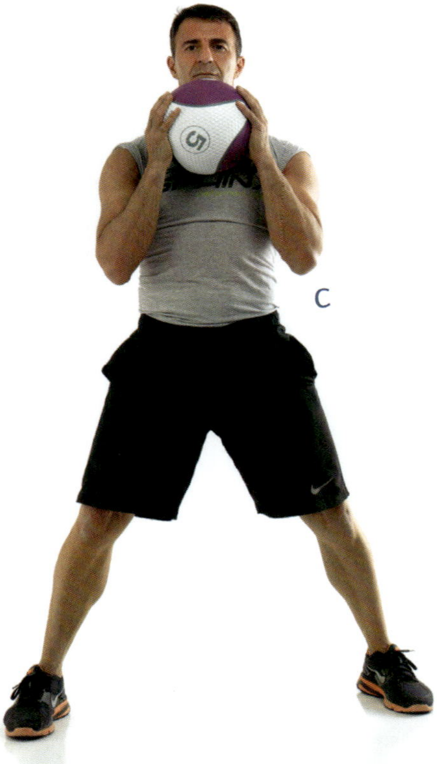

C

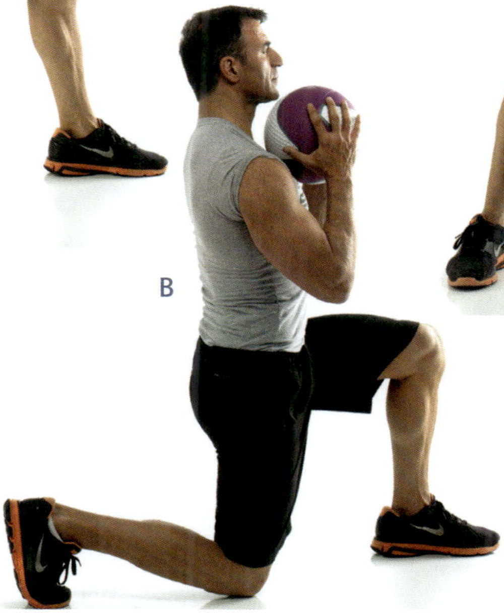

B

- **D |** Continue the rotation movement until you are in the sagittal plane again, the right leg in front of the left leg.
- **E |** Perform a lunge again, with the left knee brushing the ground. Repeat and complete the required repetitions.

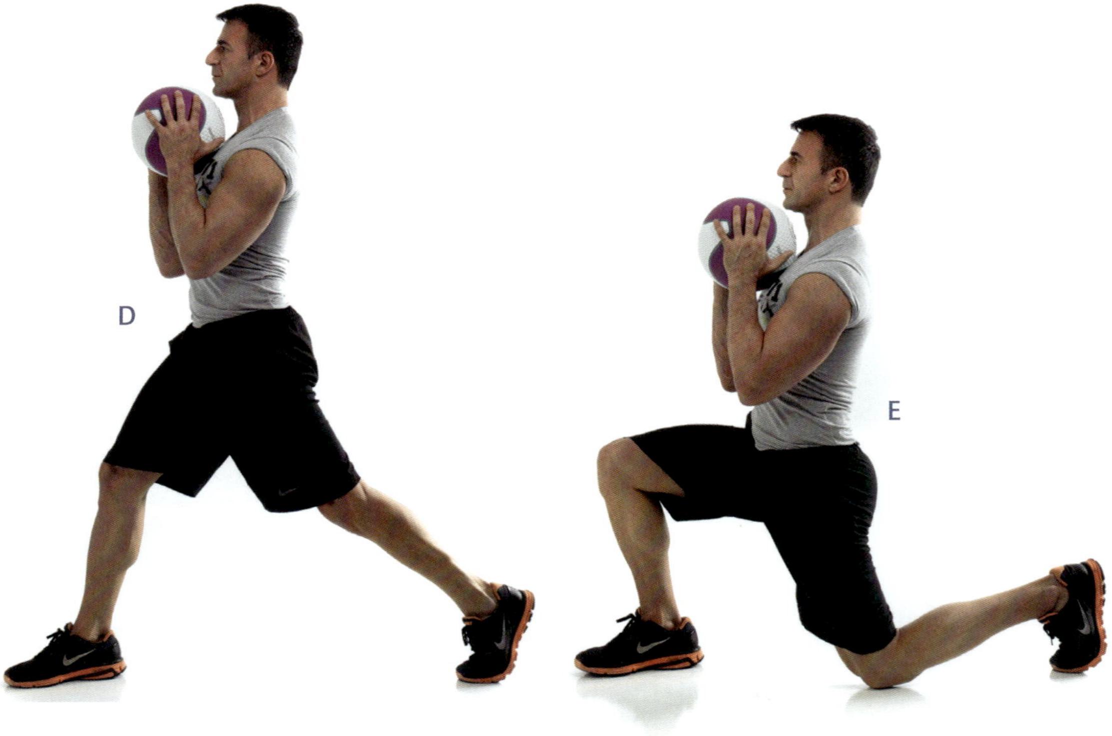

Discussion

We are familiar with the lunge movement and how the hip extensor chain is involved in it. It has many pros and few cons; it is an exercise that yields results. Body rotation and the sudden change in the movement plane are instead something new in gyms, and yet very common in performance sports, where changes of direction are a chief aspect of any game. Think about soccer, rugby, basketball, and volleyball. The beauty of this exercise is actually the synergy among the body's kinematic chains when there is a change in the movement plane: the lower bod, involving the foot, the tibial-tarsal and astragalar joint; and the abdominal fascia, back extensor muscles, and stabilizers. And significant motor skills are also involved: balance, proprioception, coordination, and spatial-temporal commutation. Truly a great exercise.

MED BALL OVERHEAD WALKING LUNGE

Starting position

- A | Stand and extend the arms above the head, bringing the med ball to the overhead position.

Execution

- B | Contract the abdomen slightly and take a step forward with the left leg.
- C | Perform a lunge.

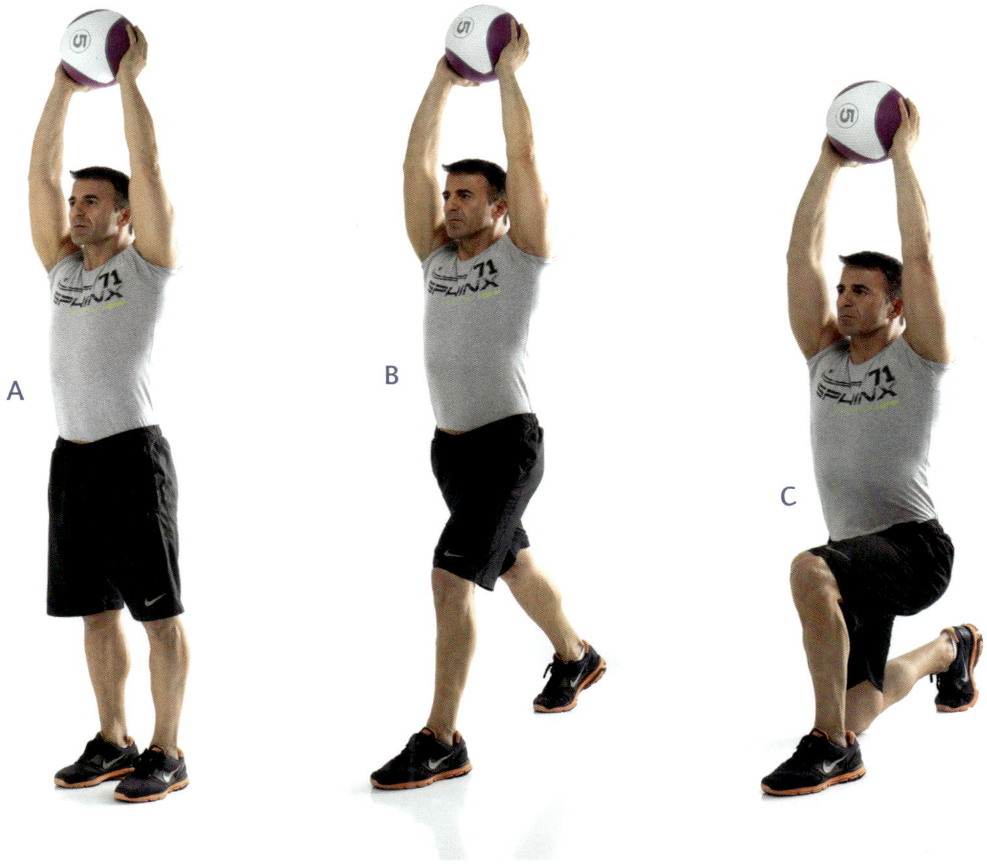

- **D |** Push the right leg up and forward, taking a step forward.
- **E |** Perform another lunge. Repeat, completing the required repetitions.

D

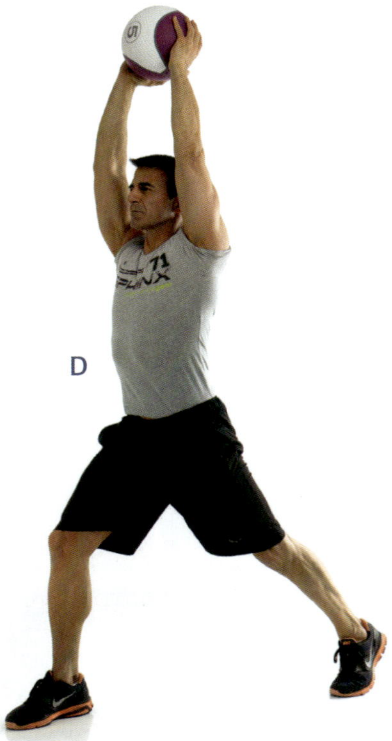

E

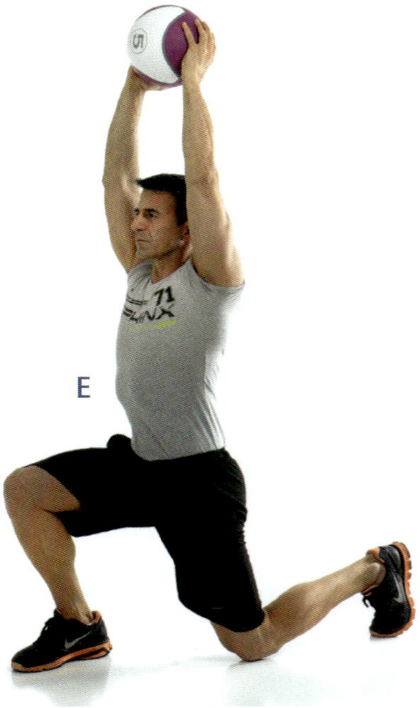

Discussion

This exercise confirms that arms are important in maintaining balance. The med ball overhead walking lunge is a great balance exercise. Let's do a roll call:

- Hip extensor chain... present.
- Abdominal fascia... present.
- Back extensor chain... present.
- Scapula stabilizers.... present.
- Humerus retractor muscles ... present.
- Proprioception... present.
- Balance... present.

They are all here! Let me only add that few athletic training programs can afford to do without this exercise.

MED BALL CROSS LUNGE

Starting position

- **A |** Stand and hold the med ball in the Zercher position.
  Take a step forward with the left leg.

Execution

- **B |** Perform a lunge.

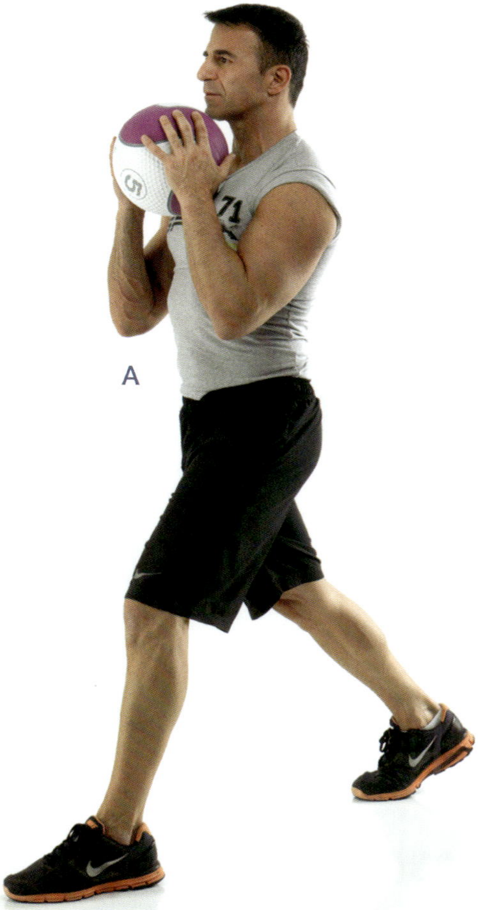

A

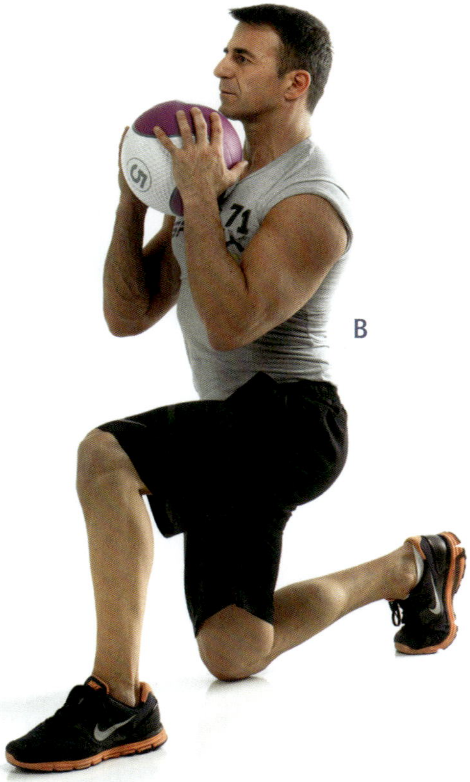

B

- C | Jump up, switching the position of the legs (right leg forward and left leg back) in midair.
- D | Land, stabilize, and perform a lunge. Finally, jump up, switching the position of the legs again (left leg forward and right leg back).

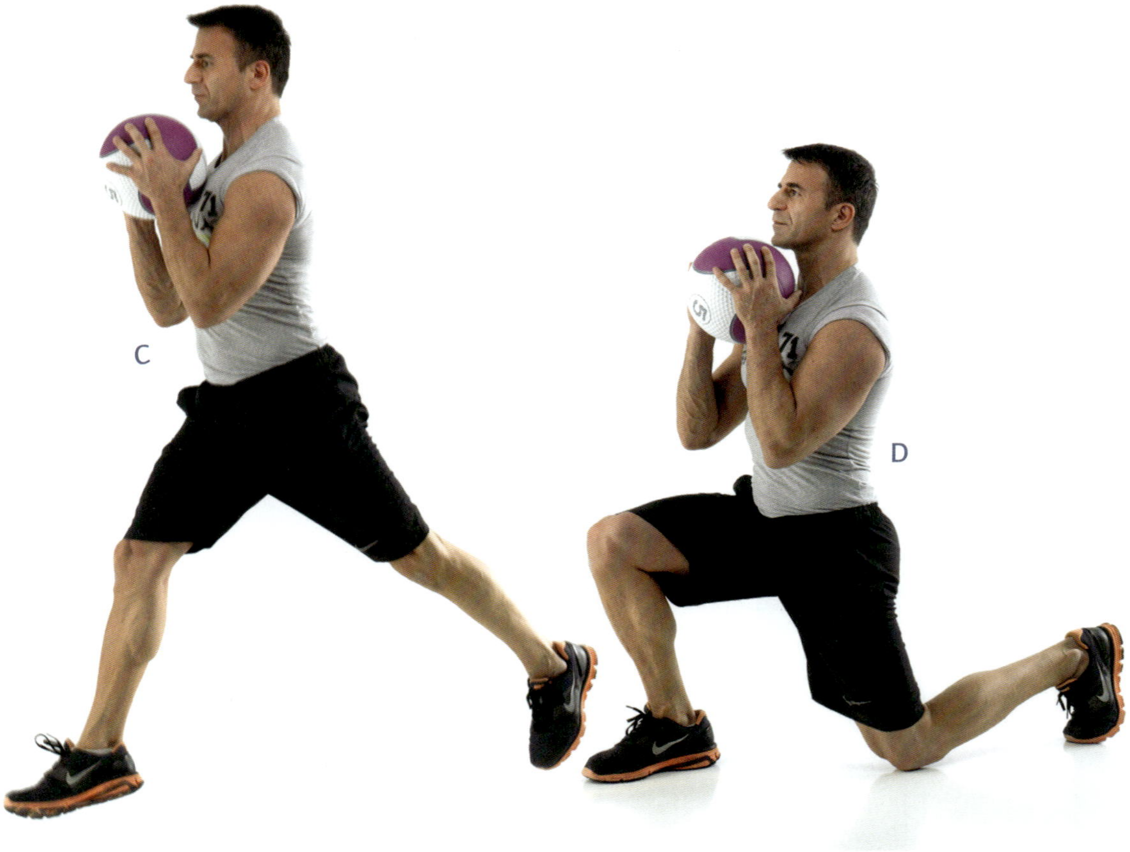

Discussion

This exercise is excellent and highly functional, suited to expert athletes. The propulsion function of the hip extensor chain is emphasized here. The exercise also requires excellent motor skills: coordination, proprioception, stabilization, and balance. The med ball lunge jump must be a part of athletic training programs for all jump and contact sports, such as basketball, baseball, handball, soccer, volleyball, and track and field. The evolution of this exercise is the plyometric lunge jump in which the stabilization phase after the jump is missing, and you fall almost directly into a lunge with the contralateral limb. This is recommended for a few subjects only.

MED BALL SIDE LUNGE WITH ROTATION

Starting position

- **A |** Adopt a half-kneeling position, with the left leg forward and the right knee resting on the ground; the torso leans slightly forward.
  Grasp a med ball with both hands on the ground in front of you, keeping the arms close to the left thigh.

Execution

- **B |** Extend your legs with an explosive movement, pivoting on the forefeet at the same time. For a second you will be in the frontal plane, with the ball at your chest.

A

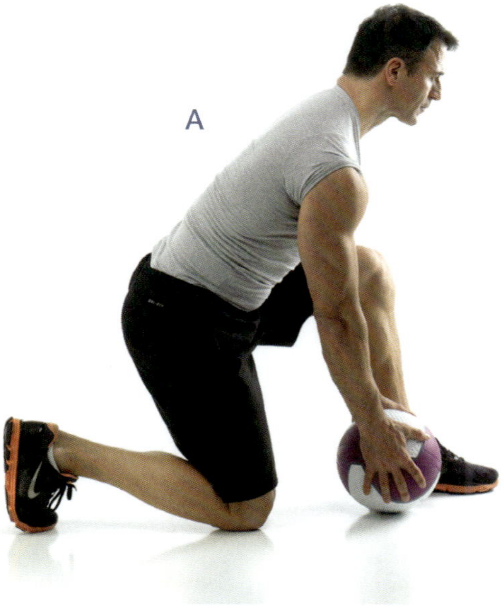

B

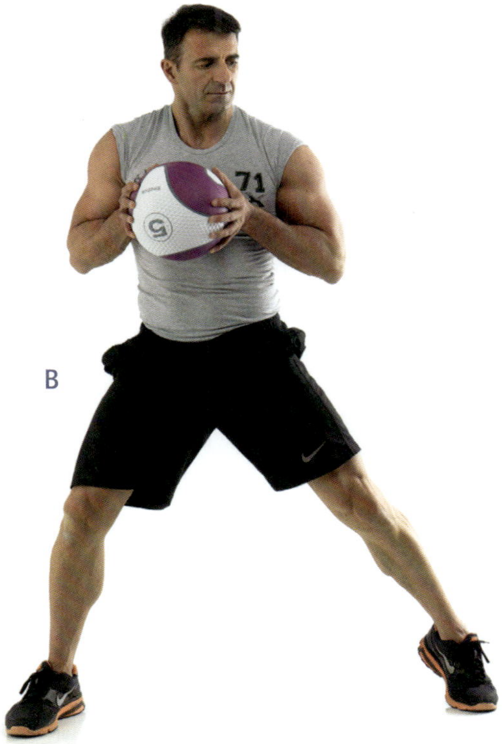

- **C |** Continue with the body's rotation, contracting the abdomen to stabilize the torso and prevent an excessive trunk rotation. Imagine you are throwing the med ball diagonally up.
- **D |** Pivoting on the forefeet, return to center, bringing the ball back to your chest. Then, with another rotation, lunge again, returning to the starting position. Complete the required repetitions and repeat on the opposite side.

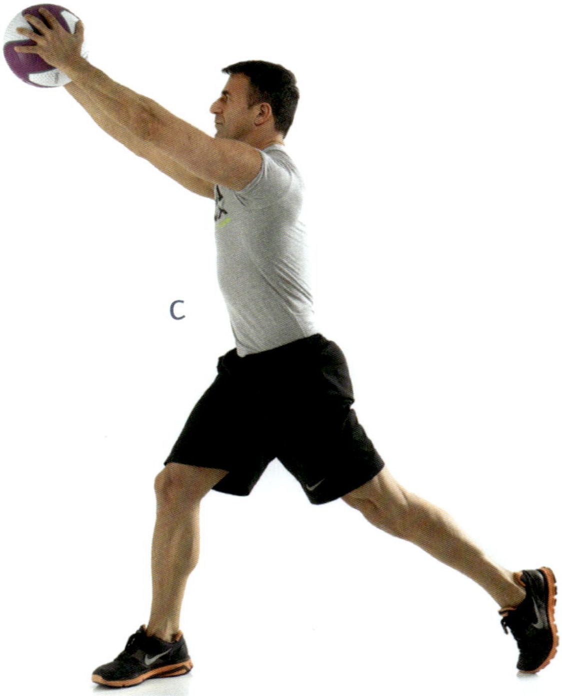

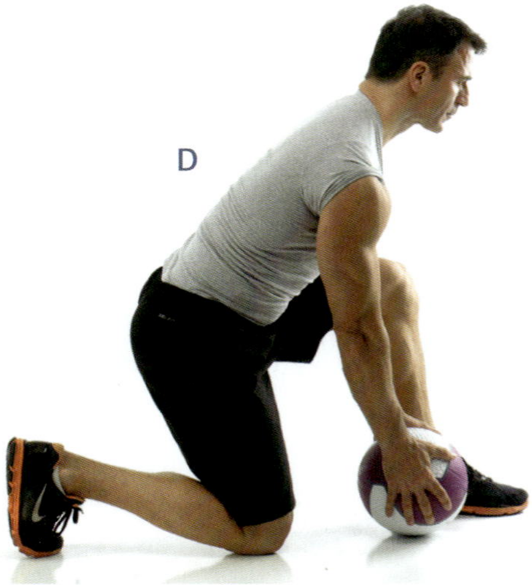

Discussion

I really love this exercise for a very simple reason: It has everything. Strength, power, coordination, balance, and proprioception. The hip extensor chain is activated in its entirety, starting from the feet's joints, which contribute significantly to propulsion. The trunk rotation movement fully stimulates the abdominal fascia, involving it both for its stabilizing and motor function (i.e., as it generates and transmits motion). The chain that relies on the scapulohumeral girdle is the center of the entire exercise. The strength imparted by the lower chain is transmitted first by the core and then by the scapulohumeral girdle to the upper body. Do you realize in how many performance sports we find this type of movement? Boxing, baseball, golf, basketball, combat arts, martial arts, wrestling, volleyball, water polo...and we could go on.

MED BALL ONE-LEG DEADLIFT

Starting position

- **A |** Stand with the med ball on the ground in front of you.
  Lift and extend the right leg slowly backward; you will be resting on the left foot only.

Execution

- **B |** Take a moment to stabilize in this position, and then lower your body forward slowly. At the same time, extend the right leg farther, while you lower your arms and grab the ball. The spine is always aligned and neutral.

A

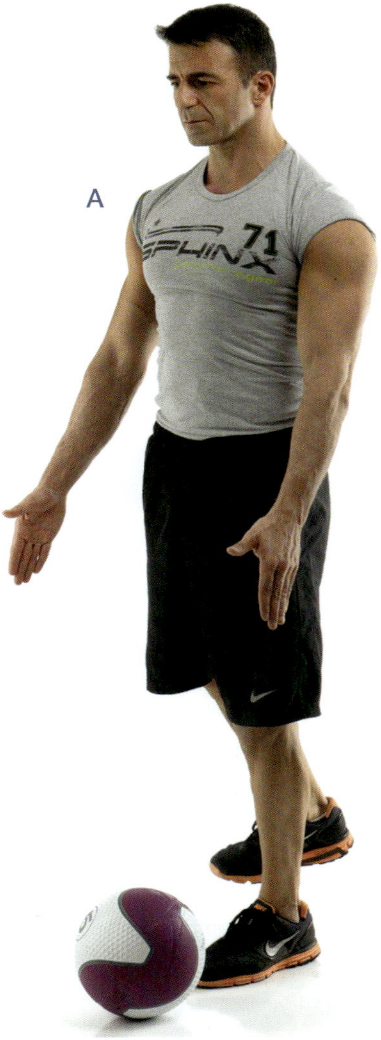

B

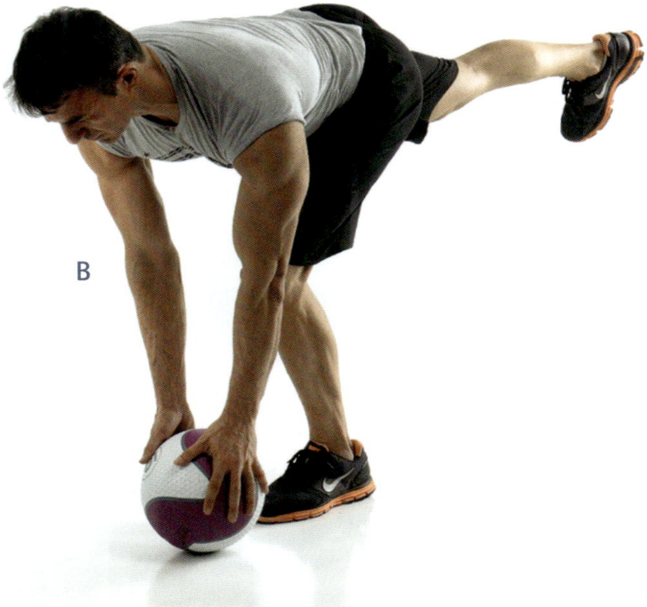

- **C |** Grasp the med ball and stand up slowly, returning to the initial position on one leg, bringing the pelvis slightly forward. Complete the repetitions and repeat with the other leg.

C

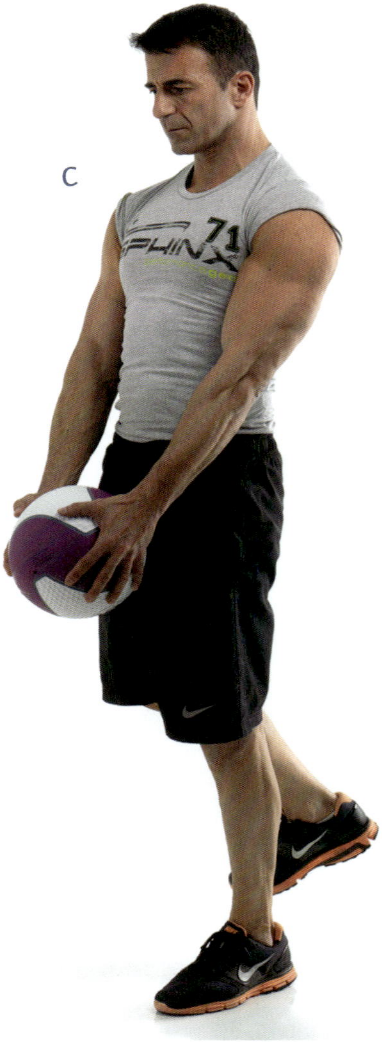

Discussion

Monopedal exercises are another of my favorite categories. The objective is to train the hip extensor chain selectively, both in the agonist part (gluteus, femoral, quadriceps, calf muscles) and the antagonist part (rectus femoris, soleus, peroneal, tibial muscles), which counterbalances the agonist part. The stress on the gluteus and the femoral biceps, in particular, is truly significant. The abdominal fascia and the entire chain of the paravertebral muscles work to stabilize the pelvis and trunk and maintain the correct neutral position. Proprioception, balance, coordination, spatial-temporal commutation, and other qualities are fully stimulated.

MED BALL DYNAMIC BOX DEADLIFT

Starting position

- **A |** Sit back in a full squat on a low-set step; the legs are apart, the spine in the neutral position (the step's height must be set for this position).
  Hold the med ball down on the ground in front of you.

A

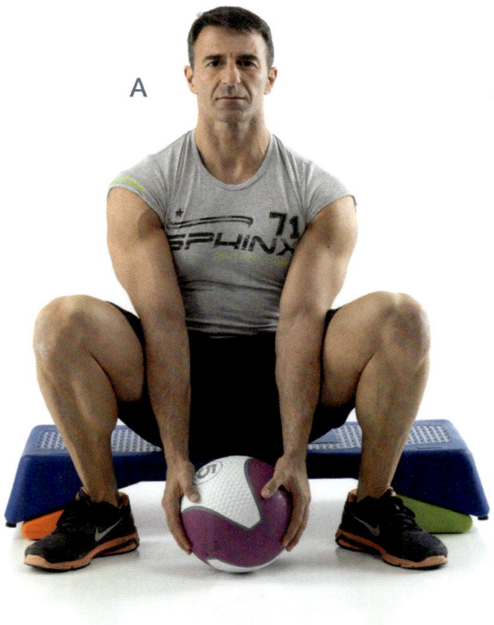

Discussion

Simple is always best. This exercise is very functional, and I am really crazy about it. Important: Try to keep the back in the neutral position from the start. Setting off from this obligatory introduction, try to bring the hips below the knees. This will ensure a strong stress on the gluteus, whereas if you stay above the knee line, it will be the quadriceps that will do most of the work. Why the step? Could we not perform the same exercise without it? Yes, we could. Actually, the dynamic deadlift is one of my favorite exercises, one of the few functional squats in which we work on function besides working on action. Yet here we have something more specific: the stop and go. When we perform a squat set, we activate a series of nerve reflexes which facilitate our movement (the myotatic reflex above all). However, if we are in a full squat position with the muscle not contracting (while we rest on the step), once we start off, the entire load is almost wholly on the gluteus. This exercise will make you work with the gluteus and the hip stabilizers (adductors) considerably and will do so even more as you progressively increase the load, progressing from a med ball to dumbbells.

Execution

- **B and C |** Stand up, explosively straightening the legs, and lift the med ball above your head. When you are halfway up, check your position. The med ball must be at chest height and the arms close to the torso. As you straighten the ball above your head, bring your head forward so as not to put stress on the cervical vertebrae. Lower the med ball and squat back down, returning to the initial position. Repeat the required repetitions.

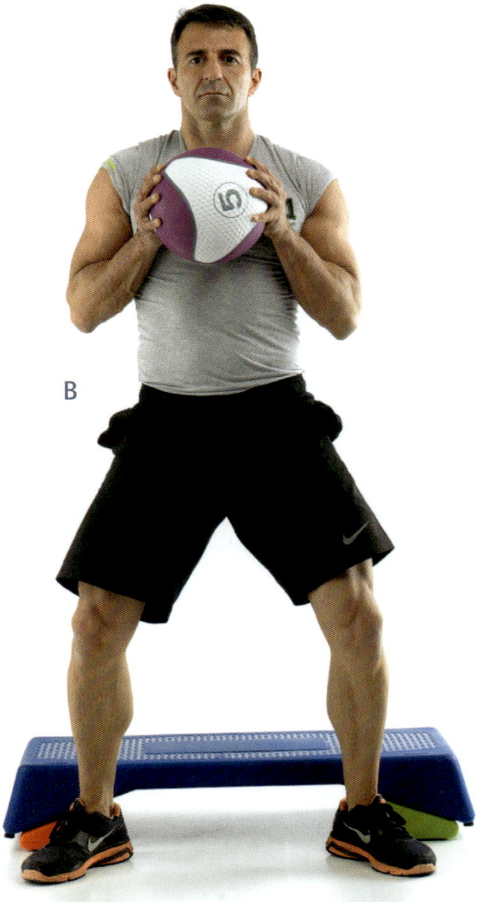

B

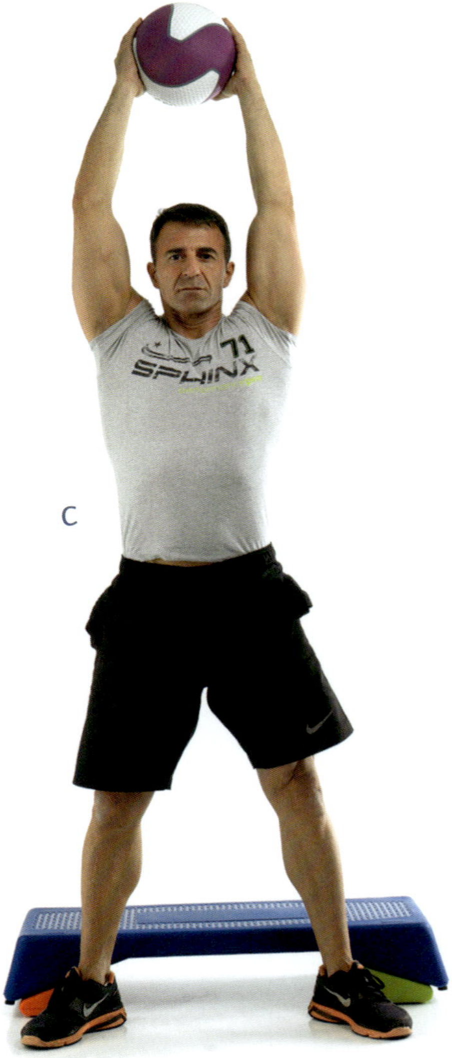

C

MED BALL SQUAT AND PRESS

Starting position

- **A |** Stand with the med ball held tightly in the Zercher position.

Execution

- **B |** Sit back into a full squat.

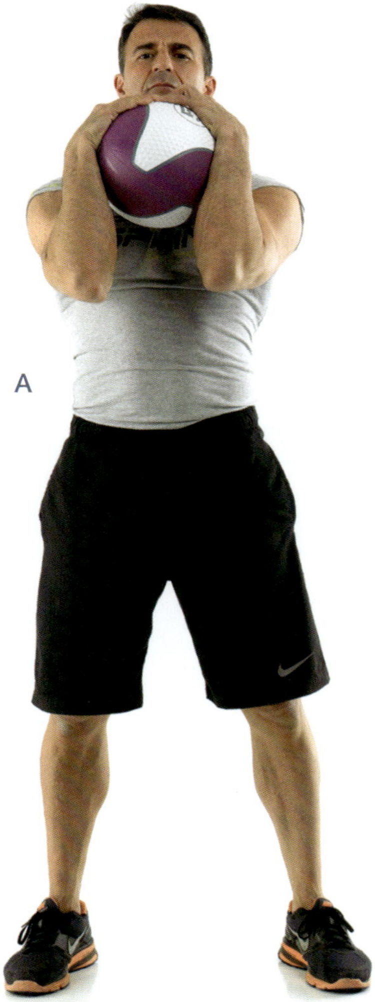

A

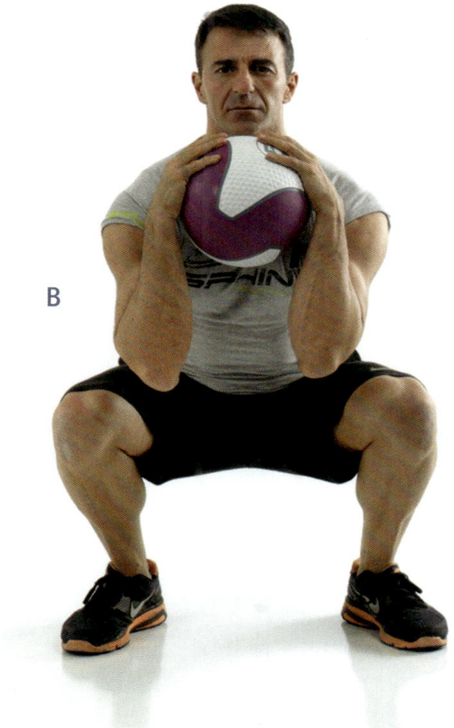

B

- C | Stand up explosively, extending the arms up and above your head. Return to the Zercher position and repeat.

C

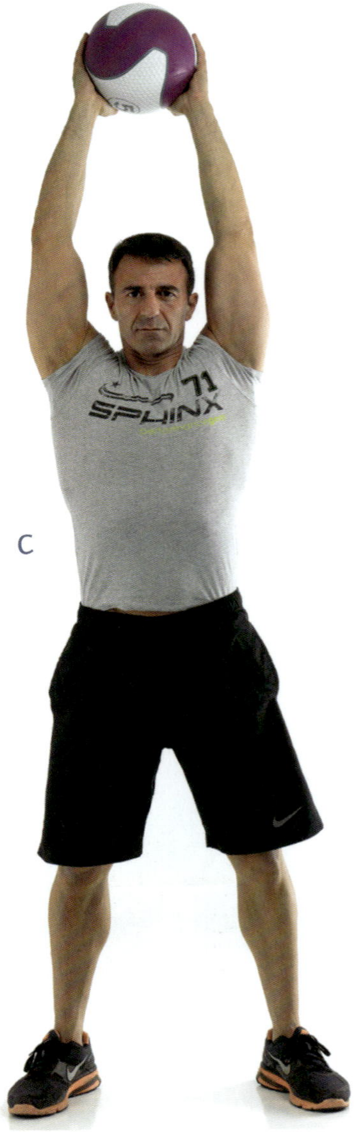

Discussion

This is a great functional exercise with many variations. For example, you can start off with a med ball or a sandbag and end up using dumbbells and barbells, and intensity will increase significantly. It is one of the few functional squats in which the flexion–extension action of the gluteus combines with its function, propulsion. A coast-to-coast exercise that works with everything, from legs to shoulders to arms.

MED BALL ONE-LEG AT-THE-SHOULDER SQUAT

Starting position

- **A |** Stand and bring the med ball to the at-the-shoulder position on the left shoulder.

Execution

- **B |** Raise your right leg and extend it slowly backward but do not put it on the ground. Give your body a few seconds to adapt to this position.

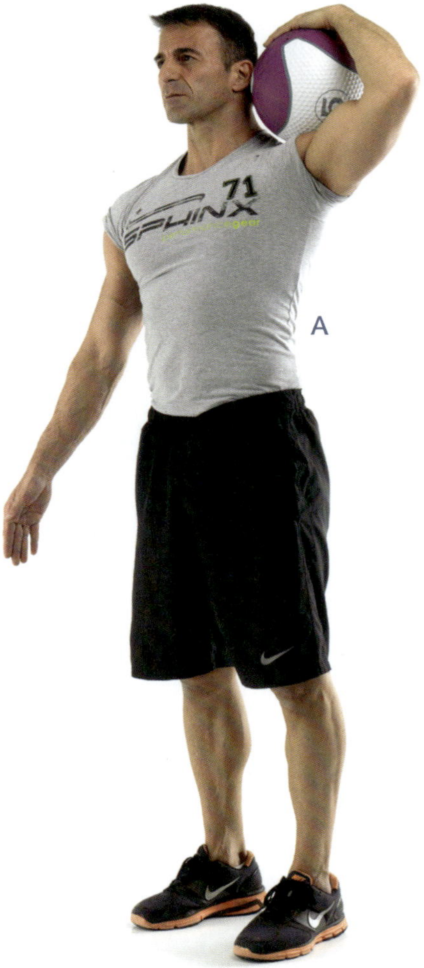

A

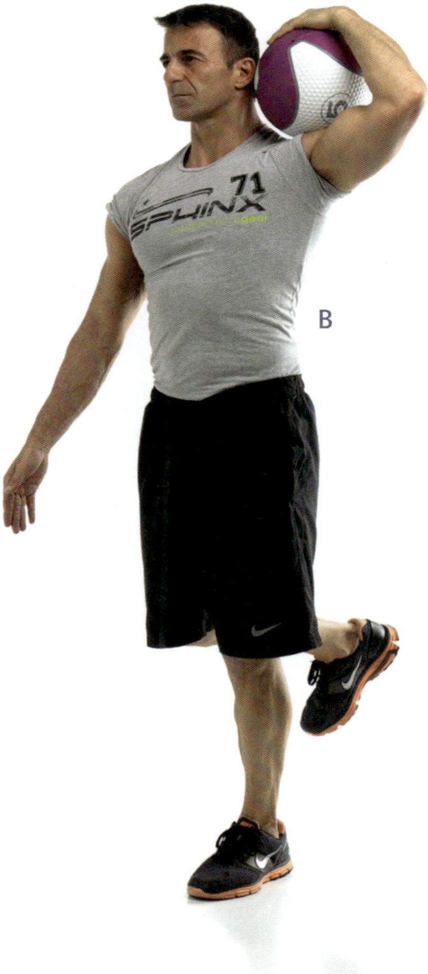

B

- **C |** Squat down slowly with the left leg, using the right arm for balance. Touch the floor with the right hand and stand up again.
- **D |** Still standing on the left leg only, complete the required repetitions. Finally, repeat with the other leg.

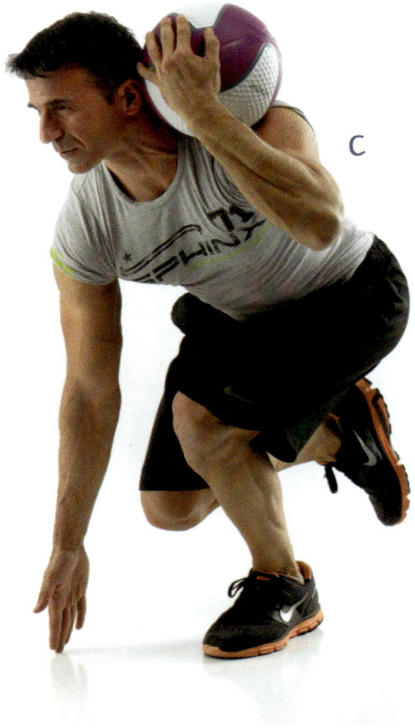

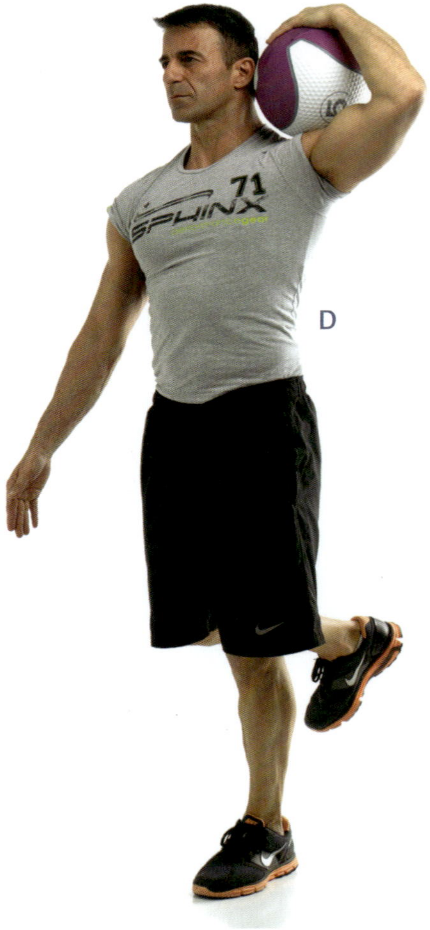

Discussion

This is another very fine exercise and, in my opinion, one of the best for the gluteus maximus. The hip and back extensor chain of both legs is stimulated by the weight of the whole body to which you add the load of the med ball or sandbag. Balance and proprioception both benefit immensely. No part of the body isn't stimulated. This is one of those classic exercises you must pass through in any advanced athletic training program.

10.3 CORE TRAINING

MED BALL ROPE CRUNCH

Starting position

- **A |** Adopt the crunch position and place a rope underneath the spine's lumbar section. Hold the med ball in your hands at chest height.

Execution

- **B |** Exhaling, lift your shoulders and try to bring your torso closer to the pelvis. Inhaling, slowly return to the starting position. Complete the required repetitions.

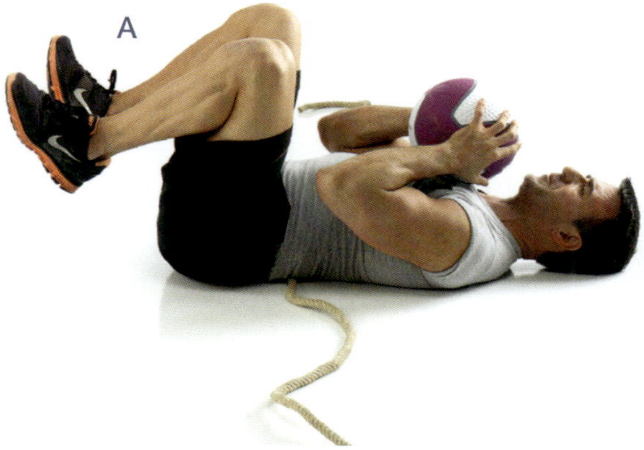

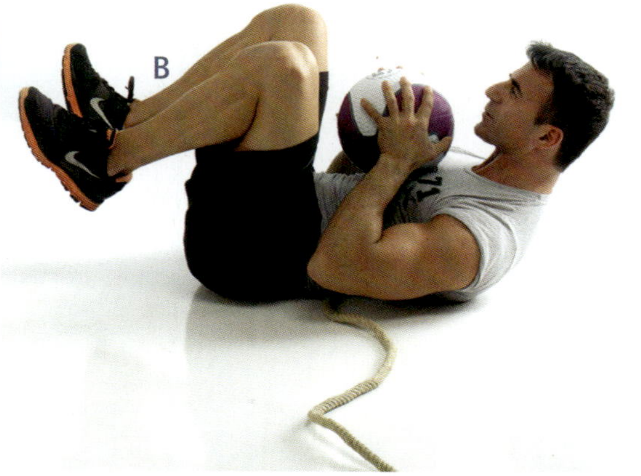

Discussion

Those who have never done a rope crunch will be surprised at how a rope placed beneath the back can change the intensity of an exercise. Michael Boyle[1], the creator of American functional training, has branded the crunch exercise as foolish and dangerous (the "Perform Better" convention, 2010, Long Beach). On the reasons why I share this judgment I have written a book (*Addominali per tutti,* Elika Publishers), which I recommend. Basically, because of the rope, we can maintain the neutral position of the spine without eliminating its physiological curves. In this manner, we will protect our back and make it less vulnerable. The med ball's load added to the rope's presence makes this crunch a great floor exercise.

---

1 Boyle M. (2010). Personal communication, *Perform Better Convention*, LA.

MED BALL PLANK

Execution

- A | Adopt the plank position, with the forearms resting on the medicine ball. Exhaling, stabilize the whole body as if it were a plank. The back is in the neutral position. Bring the ribs in slightly close to the pelvis, and push the forearms down so as to depress the scapulae.

A

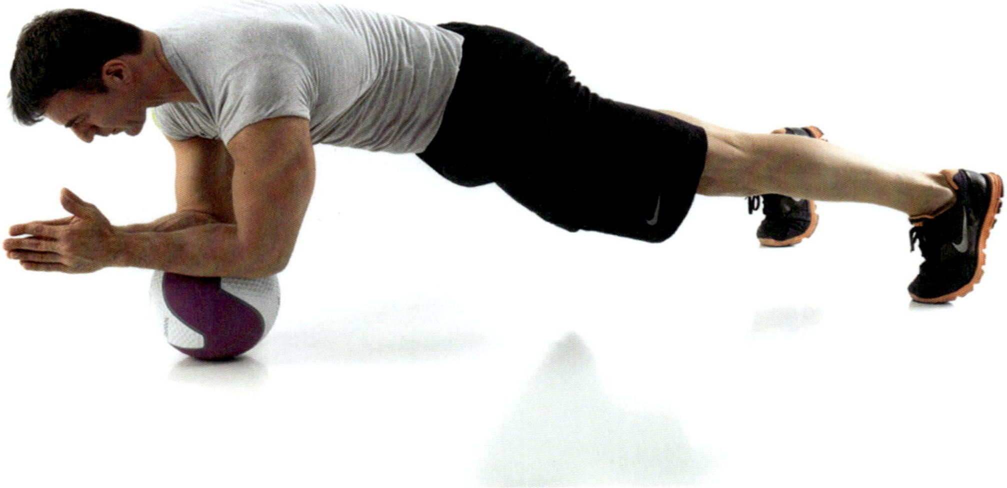

Discussion

The plank position is one of the bases of core training work (i.e., the training that works on the whole abdominal fascia). The exercise refers to the abdominal fascia's prime function: to stabilize the pelvis and torso. Furthermore, it works on the scapula stabilizers. The destabilization caused by the med ball increases the difficulty of the execution; with a hard med ball in which the surface of the ball that touches the ground is smaller, the difficulty is even greater. Start with a workout time of about 10 sec and increase progressively until you reach 1 min. You will then be ready for the next steps. There is no sport or sports fitness training, even for beginners, which ought to be done without this exercise.

ARMS-ON-SINGLE-MED BALL PLANK

Execution

- A | Adopt the plank position, with the hands on the med ball and the arms extended. Exhaling, stabilize your body as if it were a plank. Bring the ribs in slightly toward the pelvis in order to maintain the neutral spine position and depress the scapulae.
Hold the position for the preset time.

A

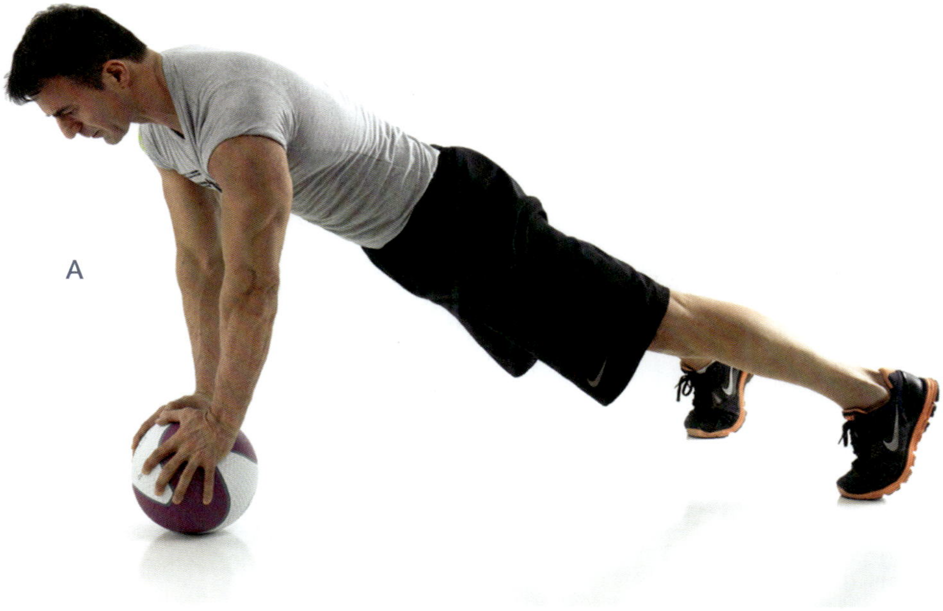

Discussion

Plank exercises are an excellent indicator of the strength of the abdominal fascia during stabilization. Do you feel burning or pain at the lumbar level? It means that your abdominal muscles have given up and the load is on the lumbar hinge. So long as the rectus abdominis—which acts as the real antagonist of the quadratus lumborum and as the lower back's protector—is working, the lumbar area will be safe, because the rectus abdominis will bear the whole workload. You will notice how much this exercise trains the stabilizer muscles of the scapula and the rotator cuff. Don't be surprised to feel the pectoralis major and latissimus dorsi, wrongly claimed to be antagonists, working in synergy. The two muscles in fact work every time the torso is suspended and semi-suspended to stabilize it.

ARMS-ON-DOUBLE-MED BALL PLANK

Execution

- A | Adopt the plank position with arms straight, the hands on two medicine balls. Exhaling, close the abdomen down fully, stabilizing the scapulae and holding the back in neutral position.
Hold the position for the preset time.

A

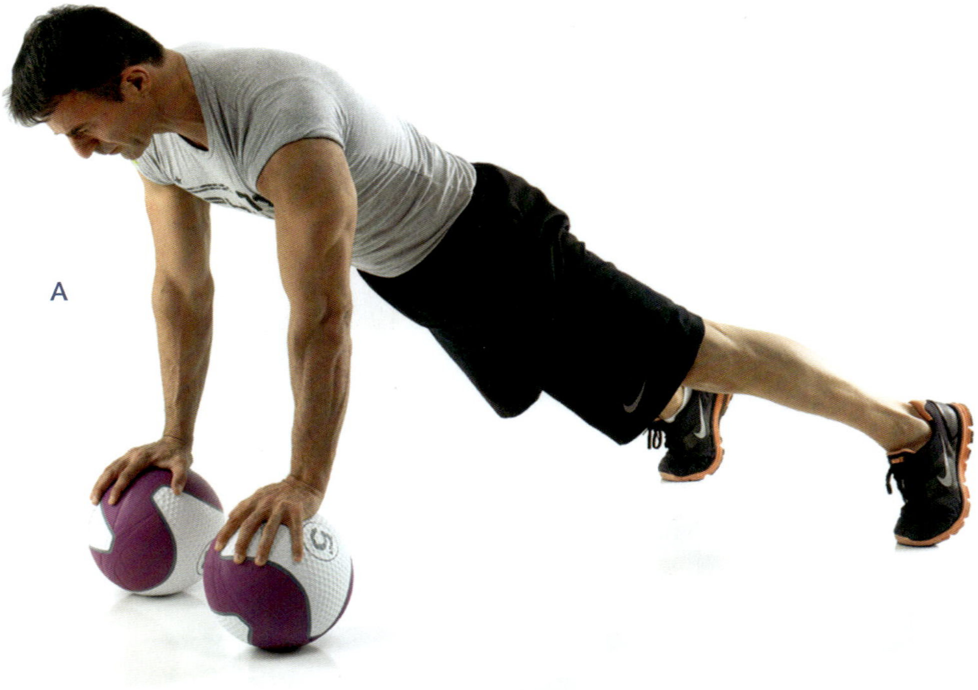

Discussion

The difficulty coefficient increases in this exercise. Stabilizing the body on two unstable med balls definitely requires more strength and control from the core and the limbs. This is a fine exercise. Here, too, the objective is to progressively increase the tension time.

MED BALLS PLANK

Execution

- **A |** Kneel on the ground, placing the forearms on two med balls set slightly apart. Extend first one leg, then the other.
  Contract the abdomen slightly, bringing the ribs closer to the pelvis. Depress and stabilize the scapulae and keep the spine in the neutral position.
  Hold the position for the preset time.

A

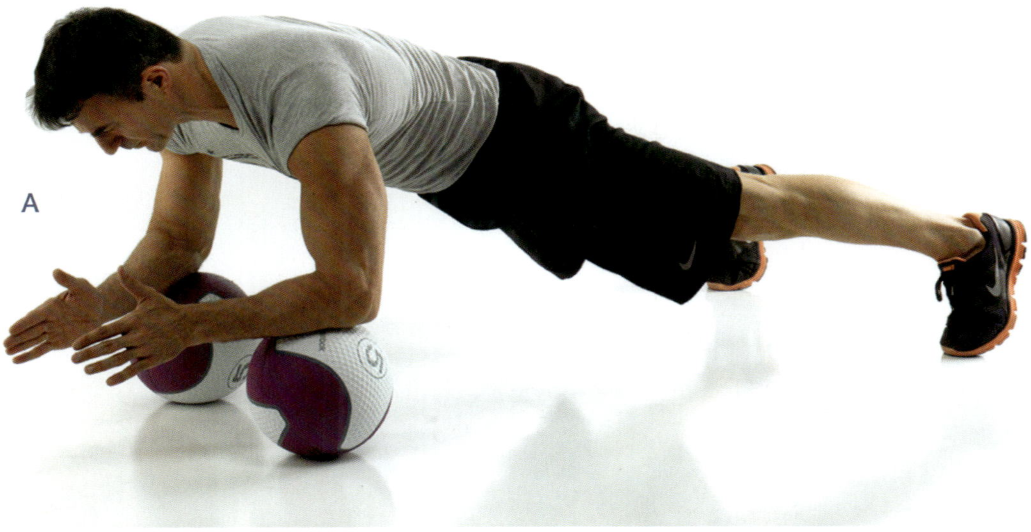

Discussion

This exercise is harder than the previous one. The presence of receptors and mechanoreceptors is greater on the palm of the hand than on the forearms, so in the straight-arm exercise there will certainly be greater recruitment. This increases the difficulty of the exercise.

MED BALL FRONT-KNEELING DYNAMIC ROTATION

Starting position

- **A |** Adopt the front-kneeling position, with the glutes raised off the heels.
  Hold a med ball in your hands, keeping the arms straight.

Execution

- **B |** Contract the abdomen slightly and turn the arms and torso to the left. You are winding up the movement.

A

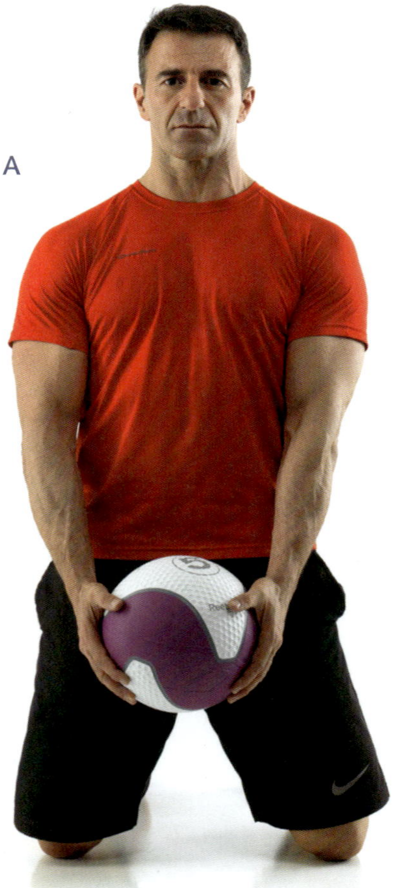

B

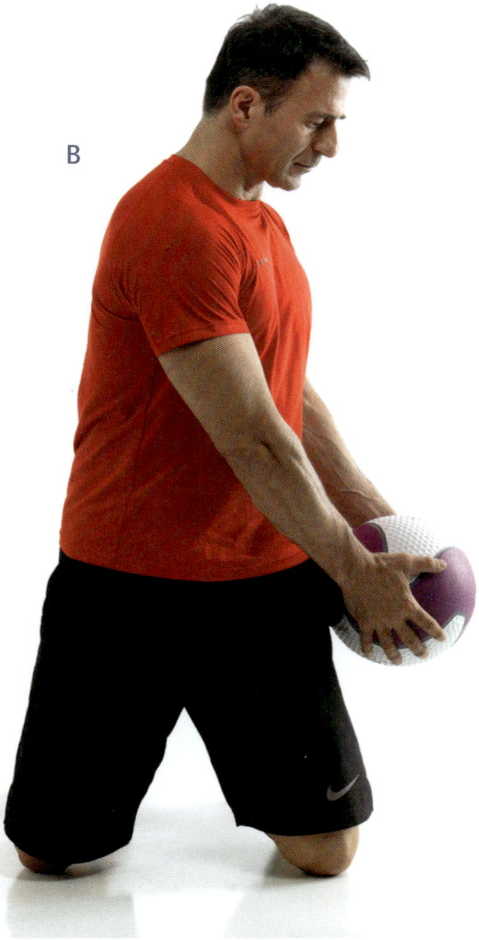

- **C |** Rotate the trunk explosively to the right, imagining you are throwing the ball with a diagonal trajectory from low to high.
- **D |** Contract the abdomen and return to the starting position. Complete the required number of repetitions.

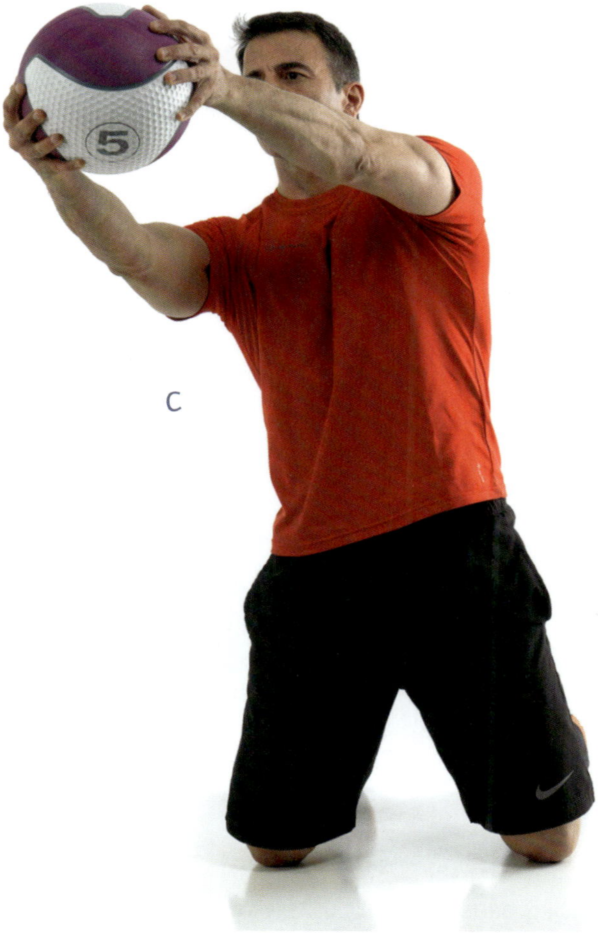

C

D

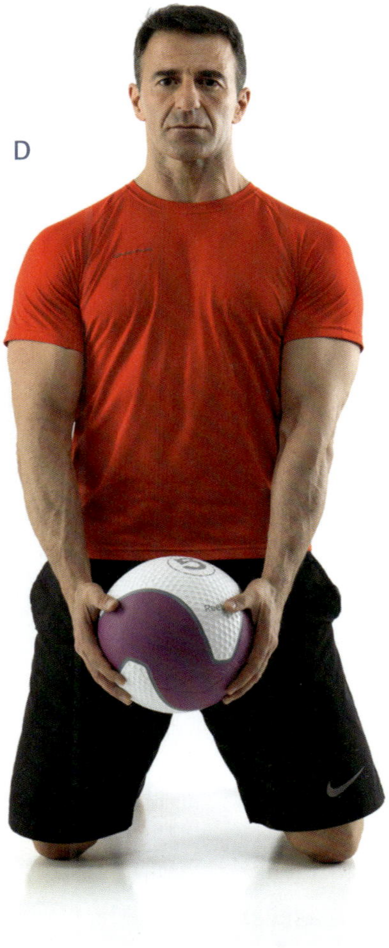

- **E and F |** Repeat on the other side.

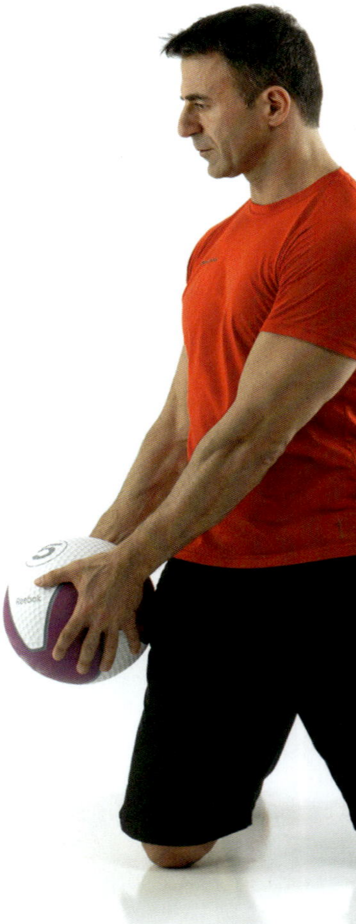

E

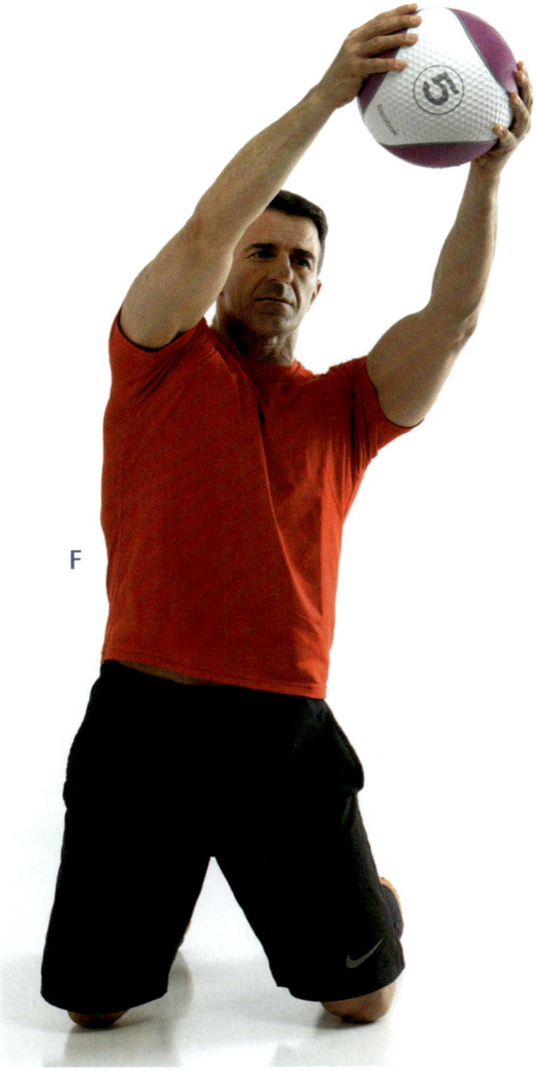

F

Discussion

This is a great exercise! The hip articular chain takes part almost exclusively with the femoral biceps and the gluteus; the core works in all its dynamic and stabilizer functions. The evolution of this exercise consists of throwing the med ball toward a wall or a partner. This is excellent for all those sports in which torsion and rotation are an active part of the performance, such as rugby, tennis, basketball, American football, combat and martial arts, judo, and MMA. It is indispensable.

MED BALL SIDE-KNEELING DYNAMIC ROTATION

Starting position

- A | Adopt the kneeling position, this time on the sagittal plane (on the side), with the glutes raised off the heels.
  Hold a med ball in your hands, with the arms straight.

Execution

- B | Contract the abdomen slightly and turn the arms and torso to the left. You are winding up the movement.

A

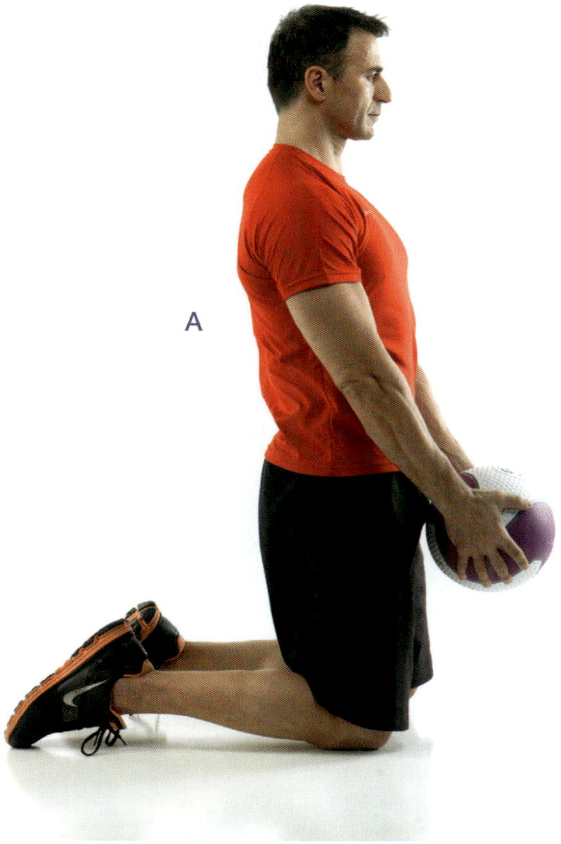

B

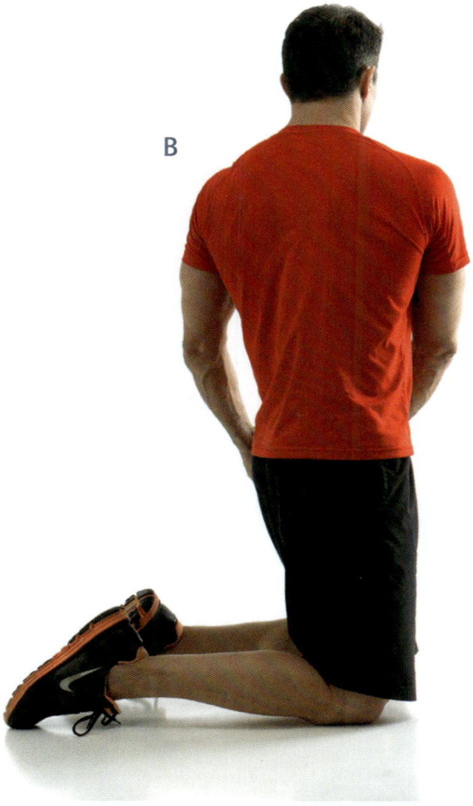

- **C |** Rotate the trunk explosively to the right, and imagine you are throwing the med ball with a diagonal trajectory from low to high.
- **D |** Contracting the abdomen, return to the starting position and complete the predetermined number of repetitions. Repeat on the other side.

C

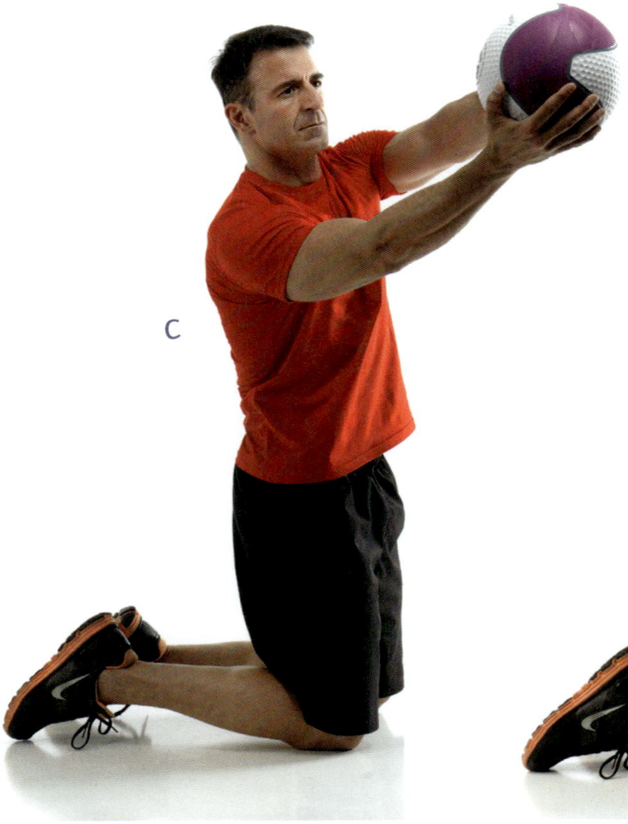

D

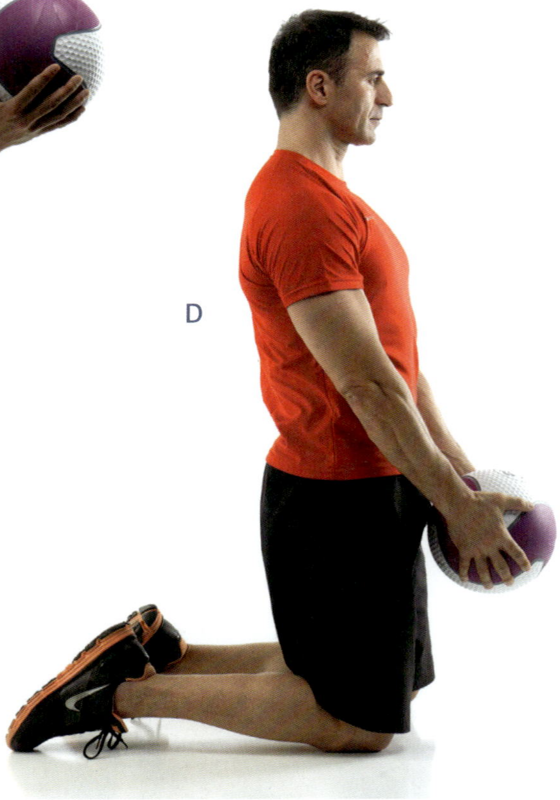

Discussion

This exercise is very similar to the previous one. What is the difference? There are many. Starting from the wind-up, which will be much greater on the sagittal plane compared to the previous movement. Acceleration is modified as a result. All this implies a greater activation of the abdominal fascia and of the muscles which support its action. Please note: When I say to imagine you are throwing the ball, the ball should actually be thrown if you are doing personal training or athletic training work.

MED BALL FRONT HALF-KNEELING DYNAMIC ROTATION

Starting position

- A | Adopt a half-kneeling position on the frontal plane: the left leg is bent, with the left foot resting on the ground; the right leg is flexed, with the knee resting on the ground. The med ball is in front of you.

Execution

- B | Grab the ball and, contracting the abdomen slightly, rotate the trunk and arms (kept straight) to the left, passing over the thigh. You are winding up the movement.

- C | Rotate the trunk explosively to the right, and imagine you are throwing the med ball with a diagonal trajectory from low to high. Contract the abdomen to return to the starting position and complete the repetitions on the same side.

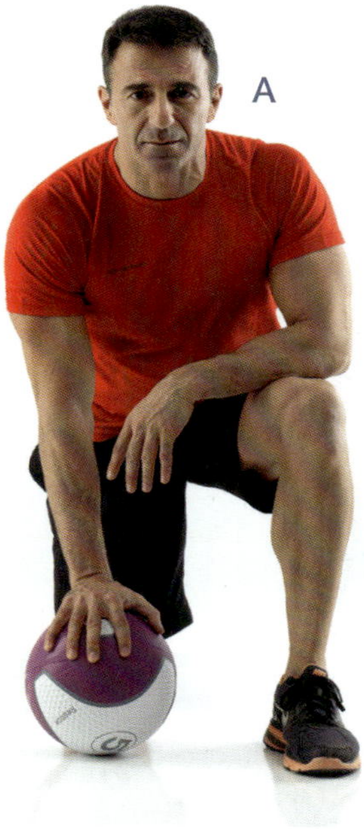

A

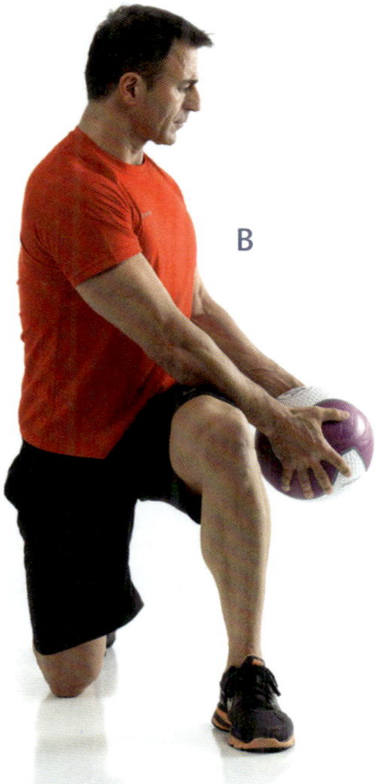

B

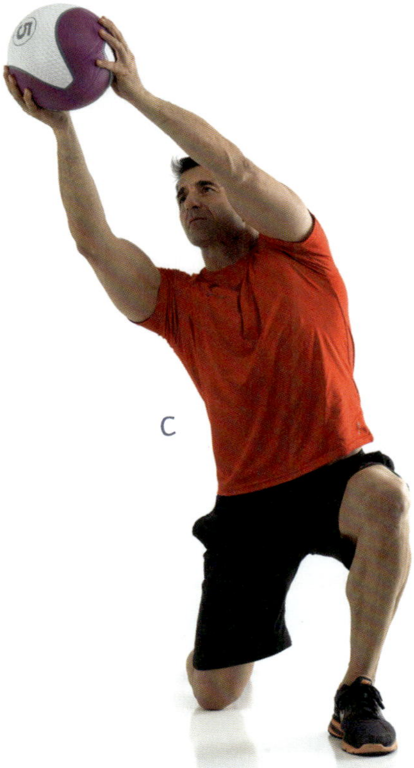

C

- **D and E |** Switch the position of the legs and execute again for the same number of repetitions.

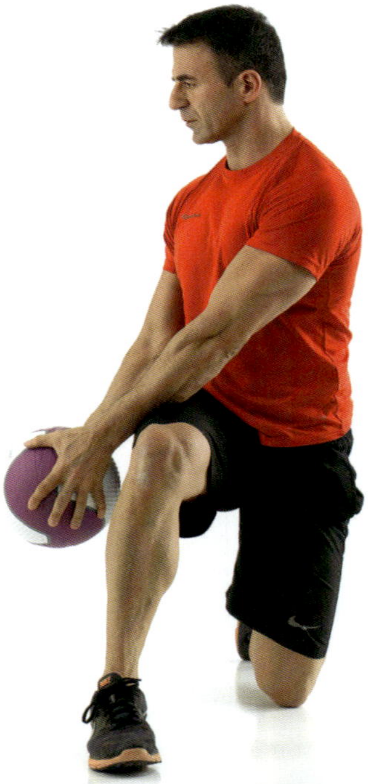

D

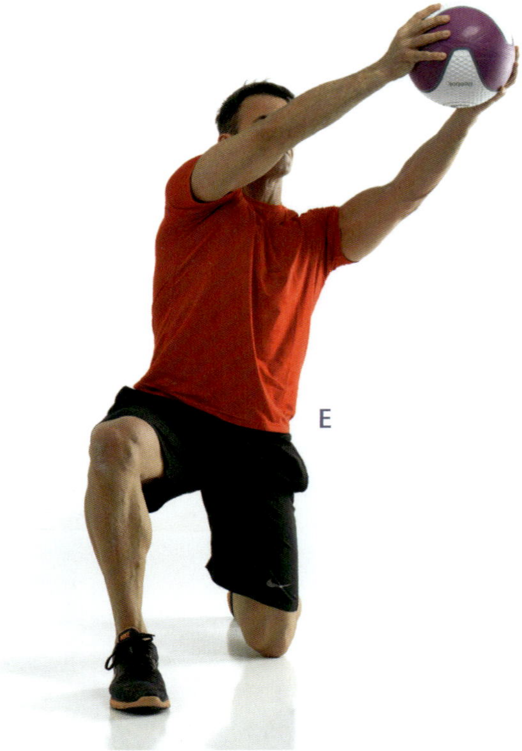

E

Discussion

Another fine, highly-functional exercise. The objective is to increase the strength of the abdominal fascia and of the musculature which supports it in dynamic torsion, rotation, flexion, and extension movements. Compared to the previous exercise, here the winding up is limited by the hip's flexing on the transverse plane (to be clear, that of the supporting foot). The intention is to deliver power and explosiveness with a limited wind-up. In this case, the progression involves the exercise becoming ballistic, throwing the med ball against a wall or toward a partner.

MED BALL SIDE HALF-KNEELING DYNAMIC ROTATION*

Starting position

- A | Adopt the half-kneeling position on the sagittal plane: the left leg is bent, the left foot resting on the ground; the right leg is flexed, the right knee resting on the ground. Grasp the med ball, contract the abdomen slightly, and rotate the trunk and arms (kept straight) to the left, passing over the thigh. You are winding up the movement.

Execution

- B | Rotate the trunk explosively to the right, and imagine you are throwing the med ball with a diagonal trajectory from low to high. Return to the starting position, contracting the abdomen, and complete the required repetitions.

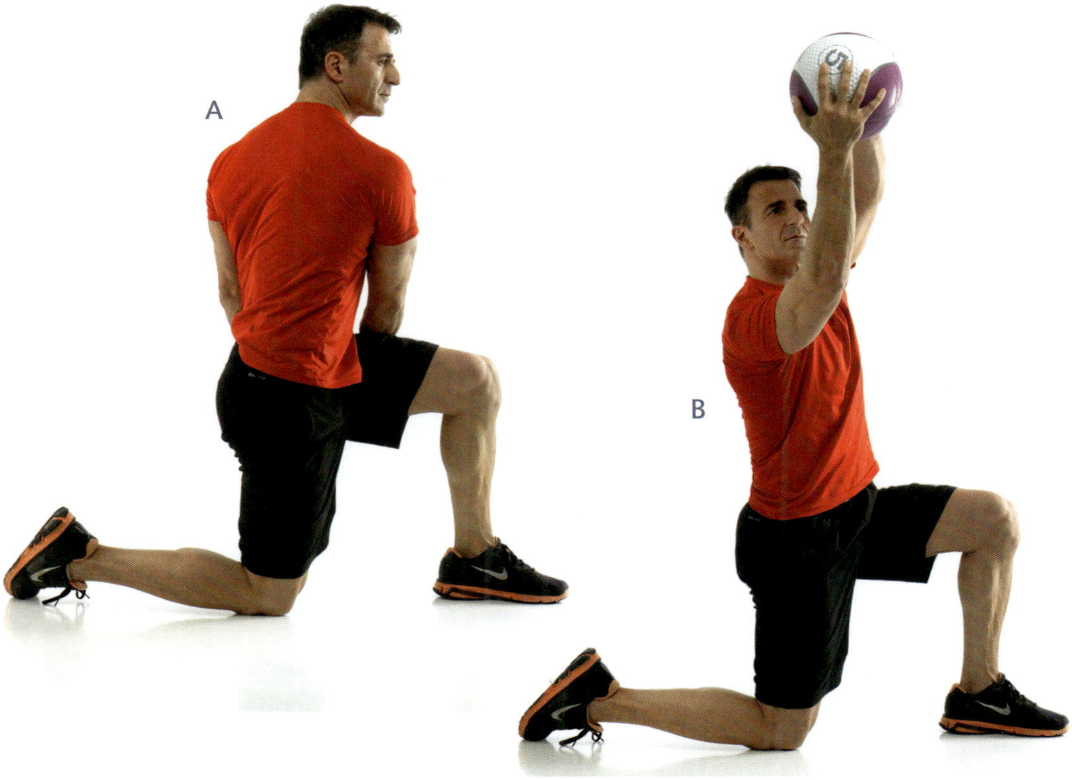

- **C and D |** Switch the position of the legs and repeat on the other side.

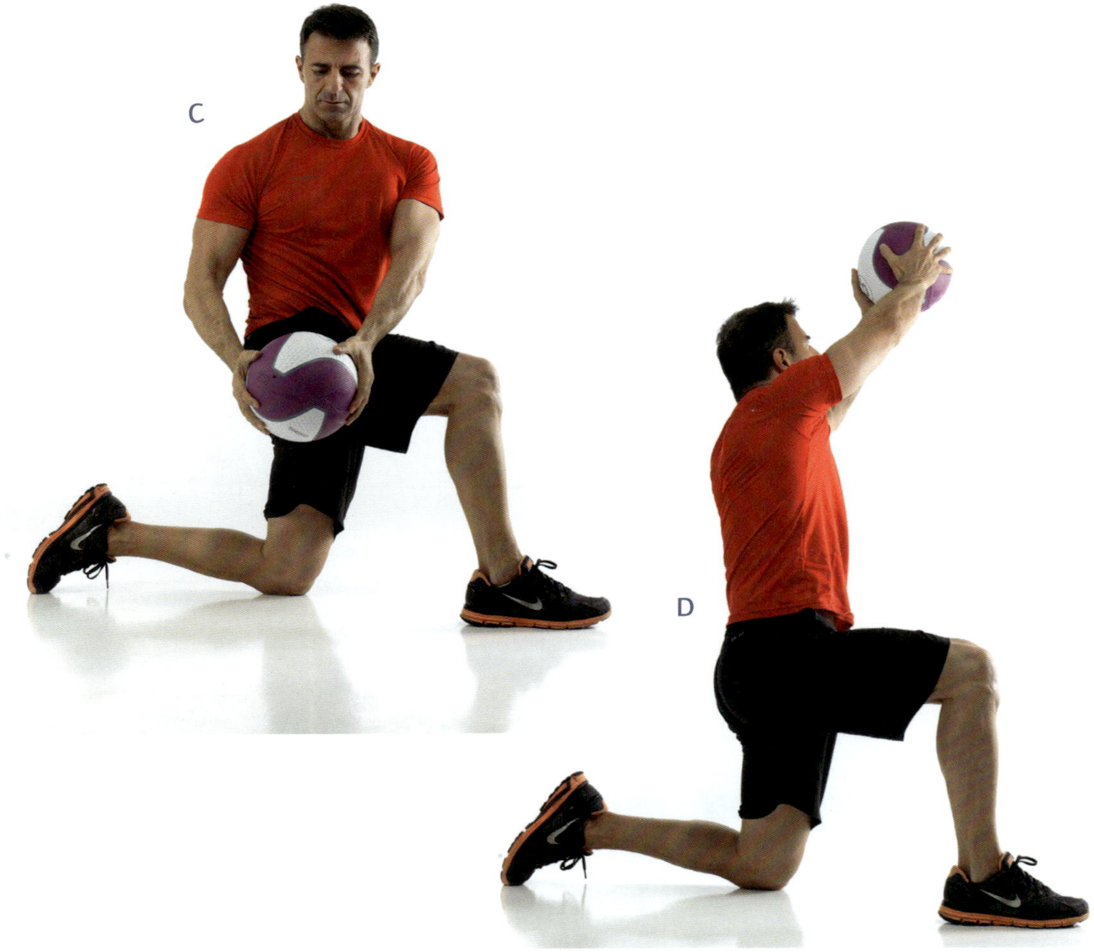

Discussion

In this case we have a greater movement range, which means greater acceleration and explosiveness, with all the related pros and cons. As for the rest, what was said for the previous exercise is the same for this exercise.

MED BALL REVERSE ROPE CRUNCH

Starting position

- **A |** Lie in the supine position, with a rope beneath the lumbar curve and the med ball between your knees.
  Close your hands into fist and place them behind the head.

A

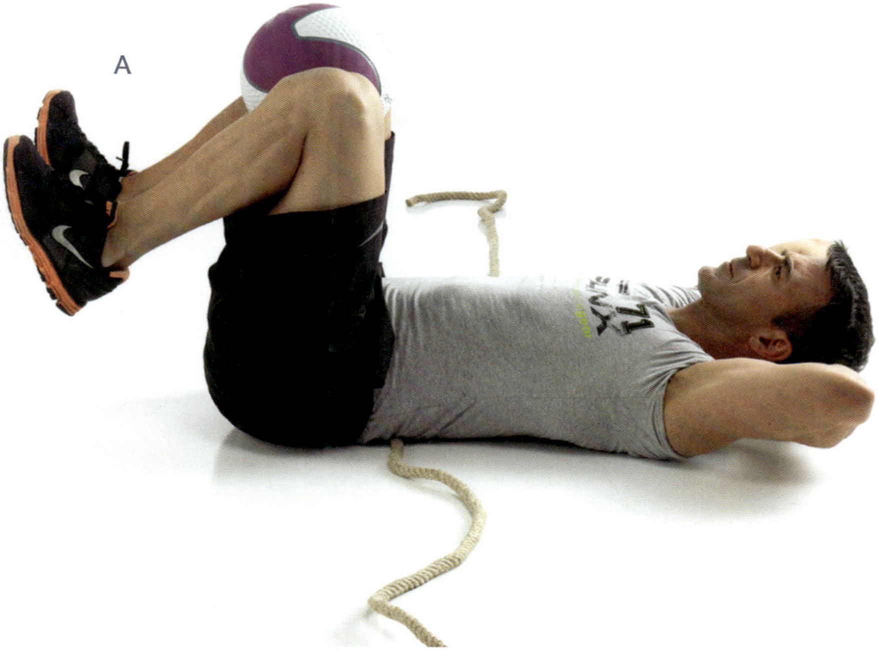

Execution

- **B |** Inhaling, squeeze the med ball tightly between your knees.
  Exhaling, flex the pelvis, and imagine you are bringing the knees toward the sternum.
  Inhaling, slowly return to the starting position.

B

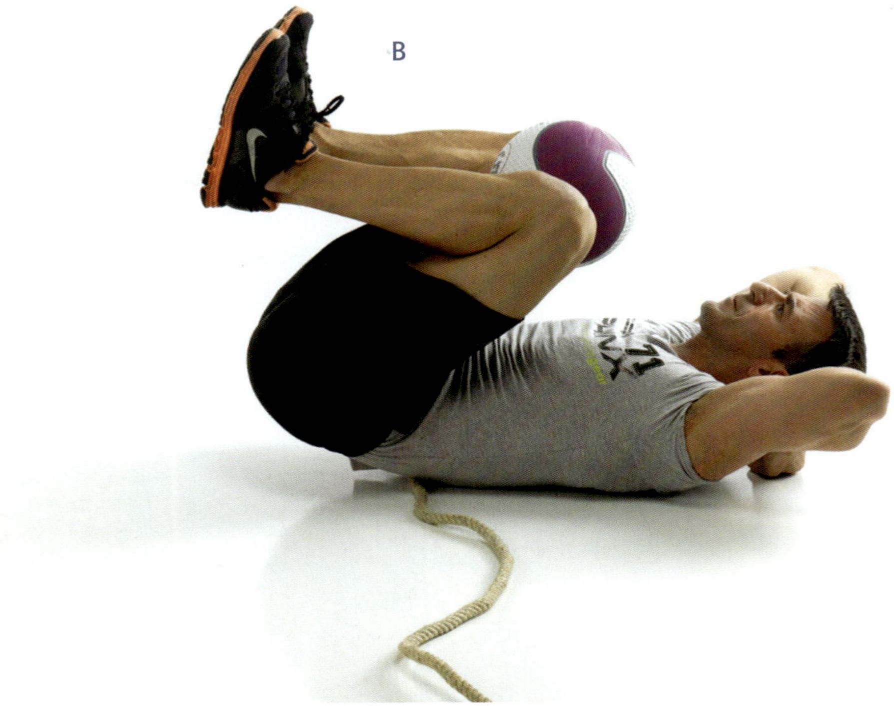

Discussion

I like all aid-free reverse crunch exercises. This is one of the few that tests the strength of the rectus abdominis. You will notice once more how much the rope's presence can change the classic exercise. Thanks to the presence of the med ball, and of course its weight, the contraction of the abdomen is really strong. Besides, the ball's stabilization, effected by the adductors, increases the stability of the pelvis and results in a greater load on the abdomen. This is a great exercise, one of the few in the crunch position for the abdominal fascia.

10.4 UPPER-BODY EXERCISES

DOUBLE MED BALL FRONT PUSH-UP

Starting position

- **A |** Adopt the quadrupedal position, with the knees on the ground and the hands resting on two med balls. Extend one leg and then the other, lifting the knees up from the ground and supporting the weight on the forefeet.

A

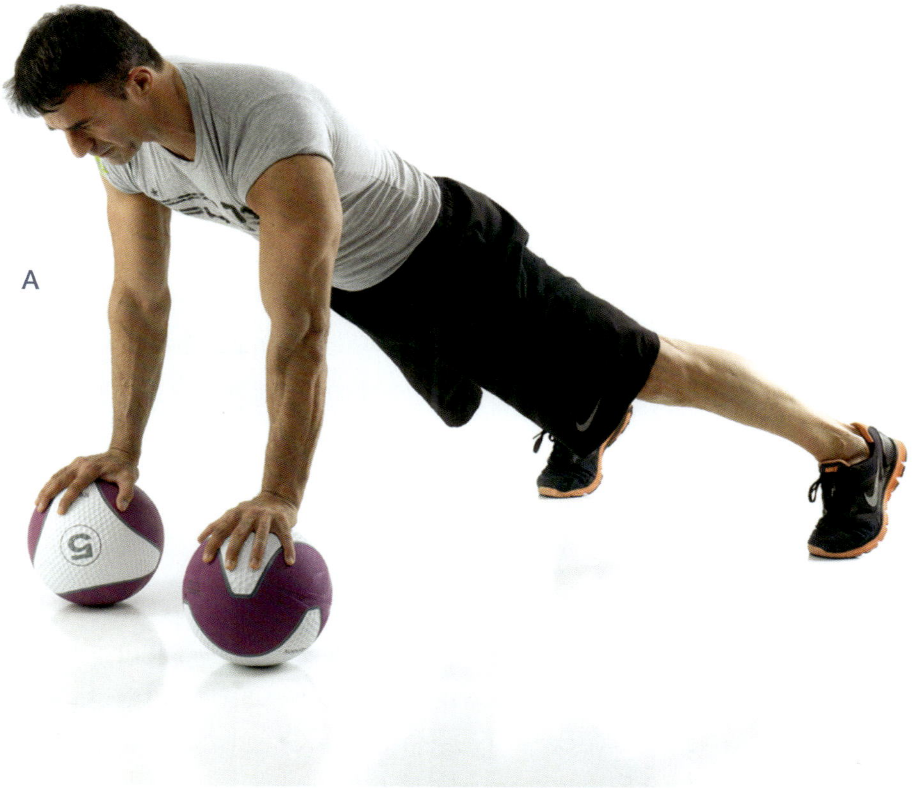

Execution

- **B |** Contract the abdomen, bringing the ribs slightly closer to the pelvis, and then bend the arms and lower the torso slowly. Try to reach below the level of the hands as they rest on the med balls. Straighten the arms, and complete the required repetitions.

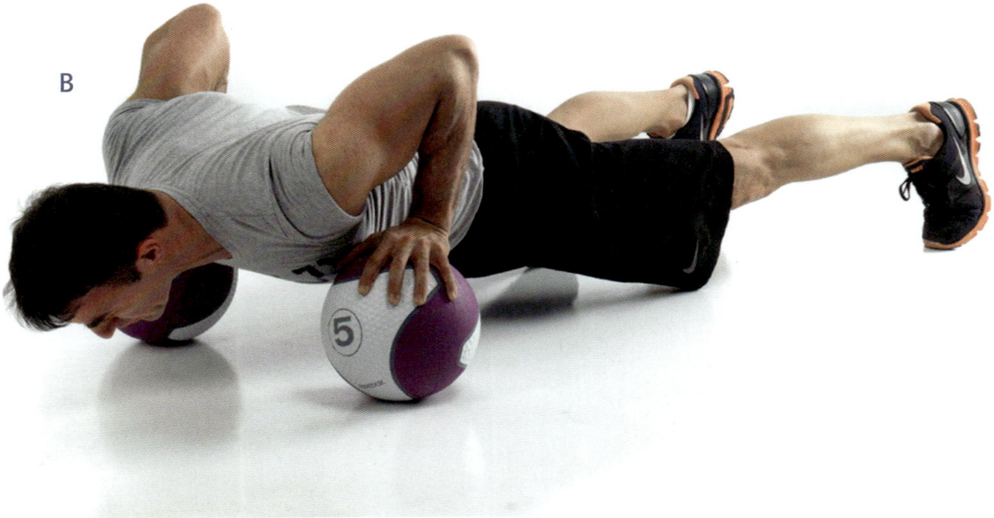
B

Discussion

For Americans, who worship push-ups, this is a cult exercise. The training of the chain that depends on the pectoralis muscles—the chest, shoulders, and triceps—is enriched by

- the destabilizing action of the two med balls;
- the involvement of the scapula and humerus stabilizers;
- the stabilizing action of the abdominal fascia; and
- the thrust phase operated by the triceps.

This is a fantastic exercise—unsuitable for beginners—that requires a significant degree of control, balance, strength, and coordination. This is no easy thing, and the exercise isn't for everyone. Our students' training path, however, involves a progression in the difficulty of the exercises to be distributed over time. Sooner or later in their sports experience they will come across this exercise. I hope they will: It means they are ready.

MED BALL CROSSOVER PUSH-UP

Starting position

- A | Adopt the quadrupedal position, with the left hand resting on the ground and the right hand on the med ball.
  Extend the legs, resting on the forefeet for support.

Execution

- B | Bend the arms and perform a push-up.

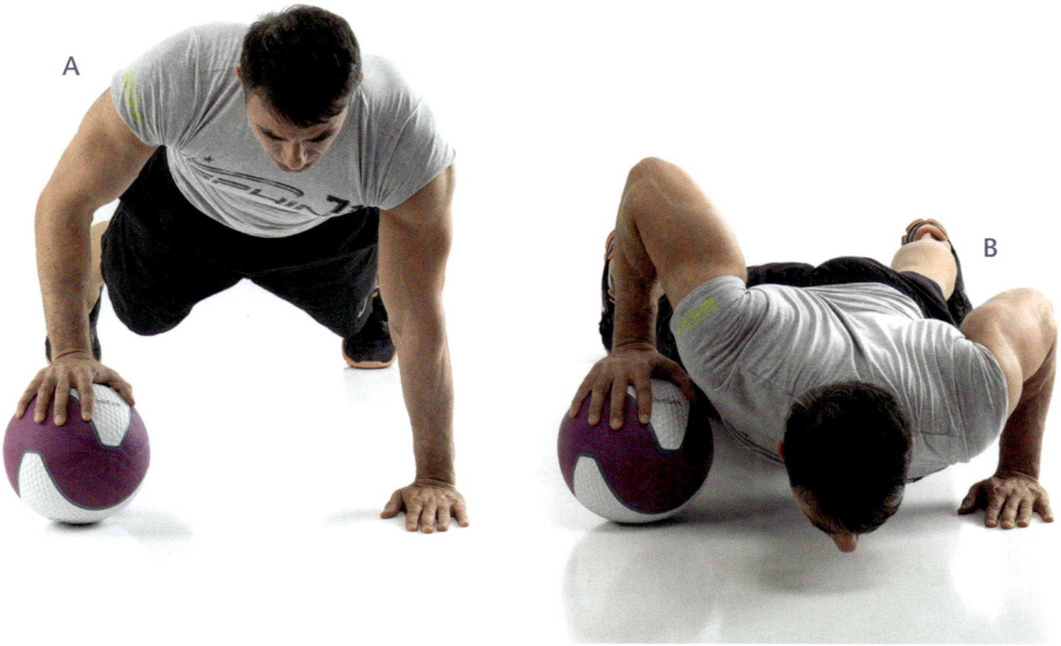

- **C |** Rise up explosively and switch the position of the hands and arms rapidly (the right hand rests on the ground, the left hand on the ball).
- **D |** Perform a push-up. Rising up, switch the position of the arms again. Continue in this manner, completing the required repetitions.

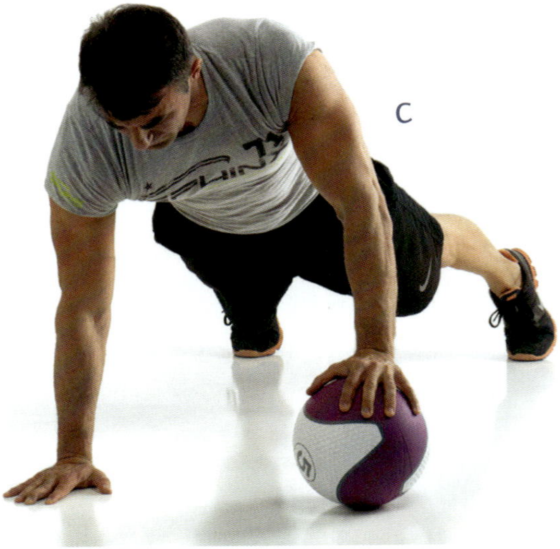

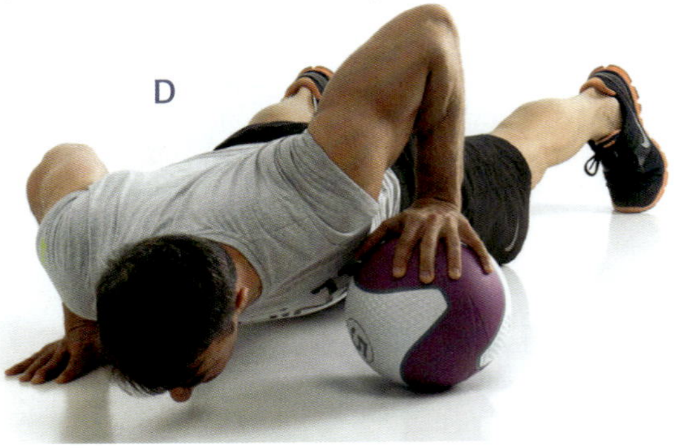

Discussion

Another cult exercise, perhaps the best-known among advanced push-ups practitioners, second only to the plyo push-up. Once again we witness a great stimulus, given the high degree of muscular stretching to the pectoralis, deltoid, triceps, rotator cuff and rhomboid muscles, and the scapula stabilizers, as well as comprehensive work in terms of proprioception, motor control, and balance. Be careful you don't spread the arms too far apart so you don't put excessive stress on the scapulohumeral girdle; the movement must be deep. This exercise is ideal for athletes who are often faced with contact situations with one or more opponents, as is the case of wrestlers, rugby players, and combat arts competition athletes. There are multiple versions of this exercise. The simplest one involves a relatively relaxed (if we may say so) shifting of the hands on the med ball from one position to the other. The most difficult version involves a plyometric, explosive transition. Circle this in red, because it really works!

MED BALL DIAMOND PUSH-UP

Starting position

- **A |** Adopt the quadrupedal position, with the knees and feet resting on the ground and the hands on the med ball. Place the hands close together so they form a diamond. Raise the knees and extend the legs.

Execution

- **B |** Find your balance without rushing, and then bend the arms in a controlled fashion and descend with the body straight as a plank, until your chest touches the ball.
Push up again, straightening the arms. Complete the required number of repetitions.

A

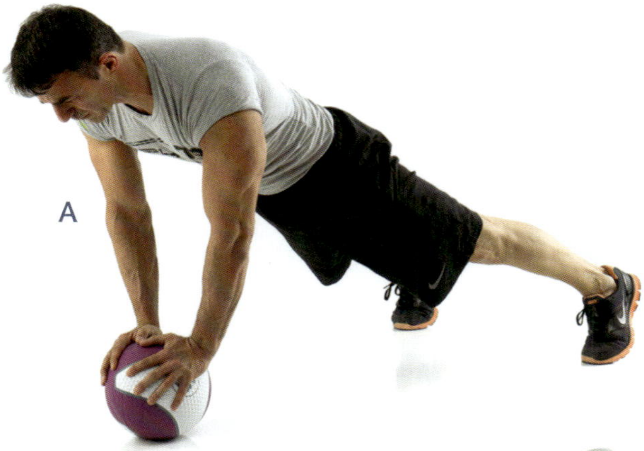

B

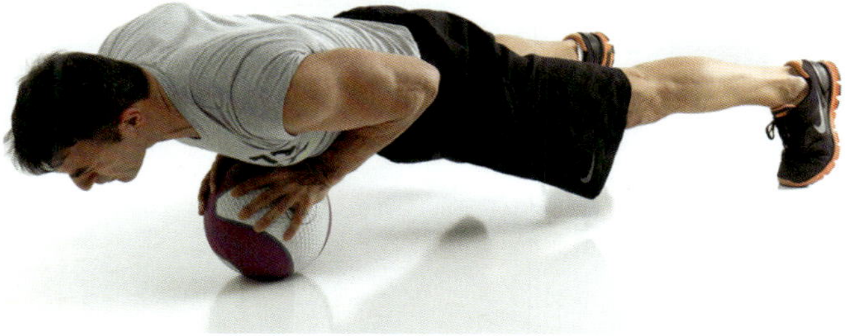

Discussion

This is a tough exercise, which stimulates the chest, shoulders, and especially the triceps. The wider-flexing of the arm on the transverse plane compared to other push-up exercises ensures greater work by the pectoralis muscle, which tires out quicker as a result of the stress to put on the triceps as extensor and retractor of the humerus. This exercise is excellent for training the weak links in the articular chain leading to the scapulohumeral girdle, which includes also the elbow, wrist, hands, and fingers joints.

HOT POTATO PUSH-UP

Starting position

- A | Adopt the push-up position, the med ball on the ground and level with your chest.

A

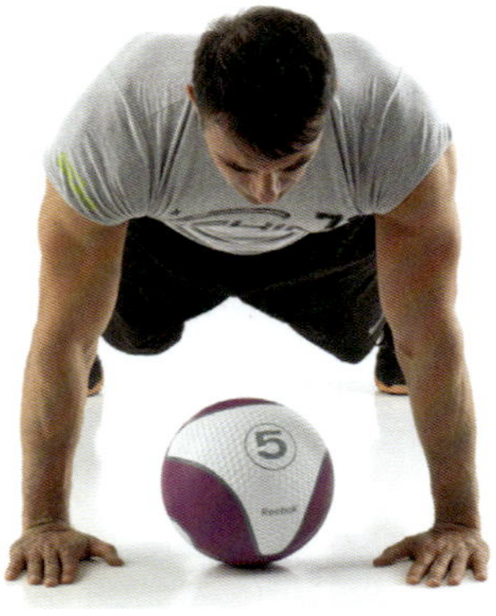

Execution

- B | Bend your arms and lower your torso until you touch the med ball with your chest.
- C | Rise up explosively, straightening the arms and briefly touching the med ball with both hands. Push off the ball with the hands slightly and return to the starting position. Start all over again.

C

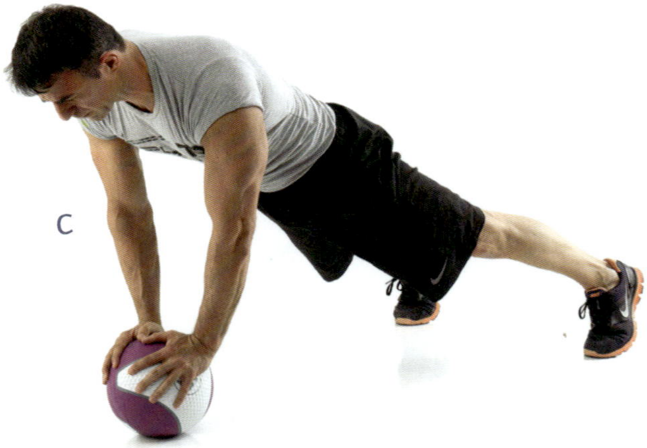

B

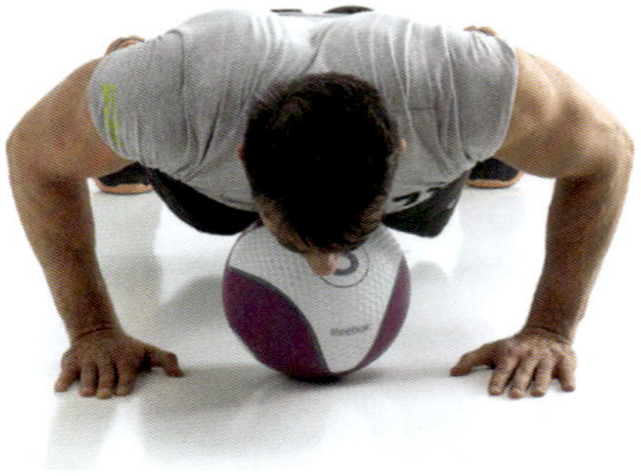

Discussion

What an exercise! The hot potato push-up is a plyometric exercise. An exercise suitable to only a few people and only for a short time, it will make a difference if the development of strength and hypertrophy of the pectoralis chain has plateaued. It works on all the weak links in the pectoralis chain, strengthening them. Besides, as all plyometric exercises do, it increases the spatial and temporal recruitment ability of the central nervous system. Not often, but do pick it out sometimes from your store of unconventional exercises.

MED BALL PLYO BENCH PRESS

Starting position

- **A |** Lie in the supine position, with the legs bent and the feet on the ground.
  Grasp the med ball and bring it to your chest.

Execution

- **B |** Throw the med ball explosively up above your body.

A

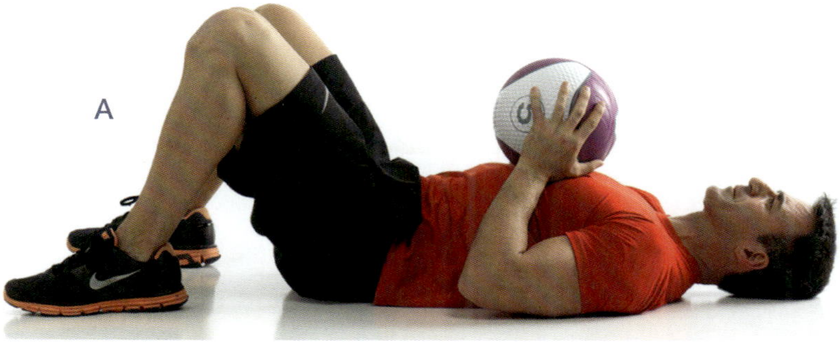

B

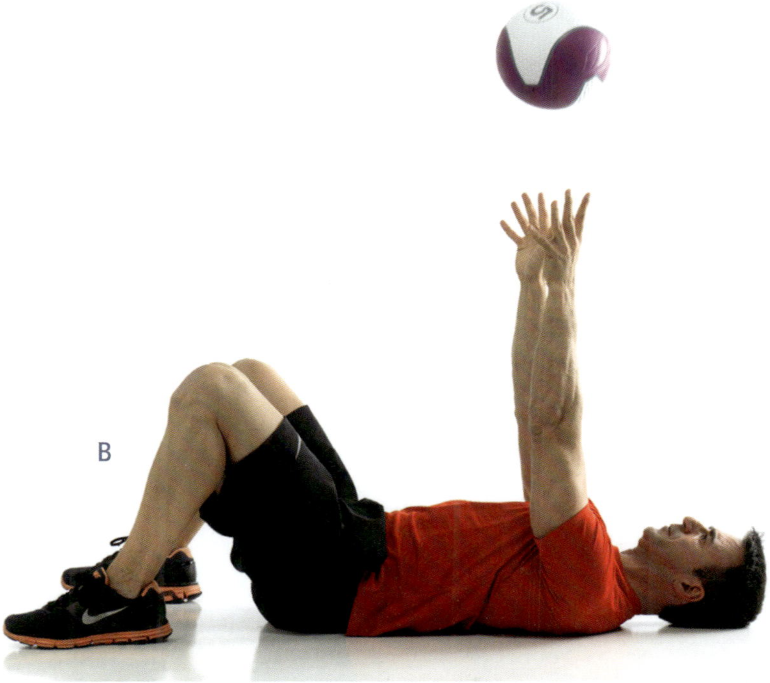

- **C |** Stay with arms half-flexed, waiting for the ball to fall.
- **D |** As soon as you catch the ball, use elastic force to explosively throw it up again. Complete the required repetitions.

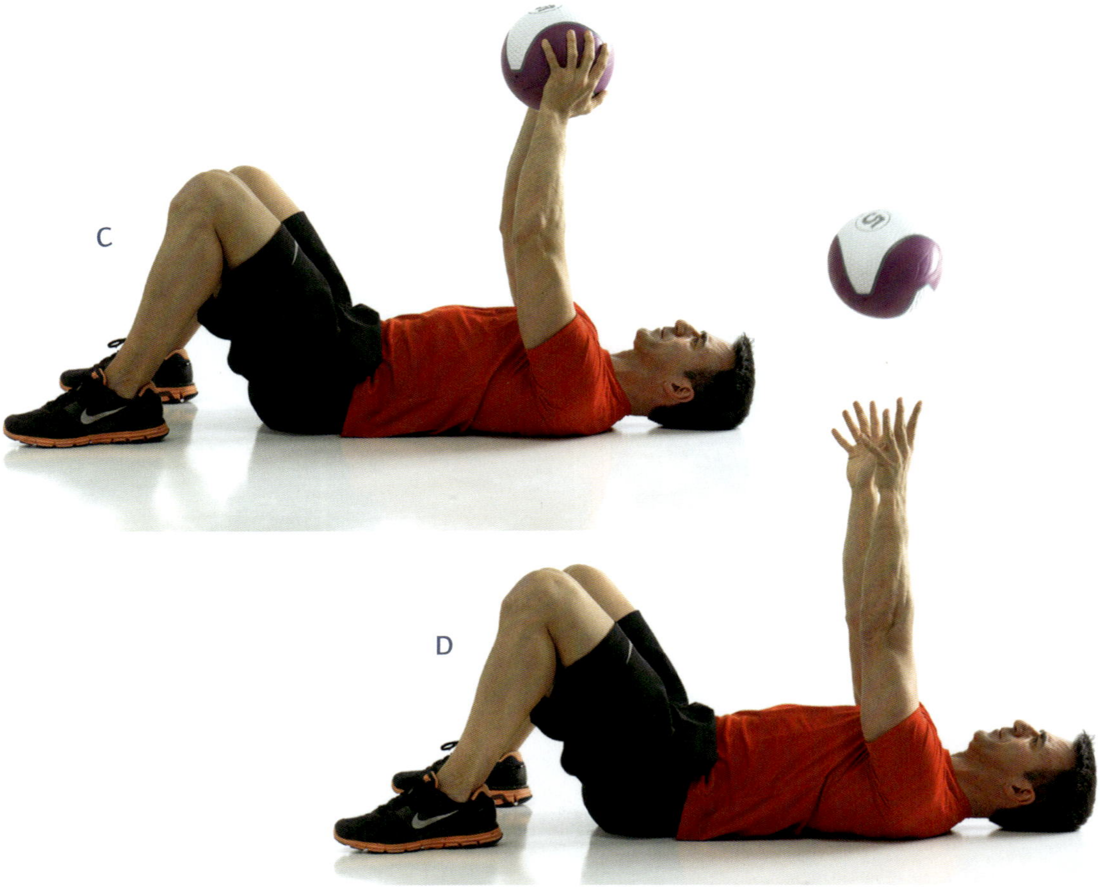

Discussion

This exercise has two versions. The simplest is the one shown. The most difficult one involves the presence of a partner standing on a bench behind you; there must be at least a 1 m (1.09 yd) differential, though the med ball's weight will influence height and performance. The first variation is an introduction to the second. Plyometric exercises increase strength and power. According to the Russian school, no training program can do without them, provided they are executed properly and in the correct amount. This may be a problem, since very often they are included almost randomly in training and athletic programs.

MED BALL DIAGONAL PRESS

Starting position

- A | Stand with the med ball in the Zercher position.

Execution

- B | Quickly bend your legs.
- C | Press the ball up diagonally to the left. The torso follows the med ball's movement and leans laterally, assisting the arms in the upward thrust.

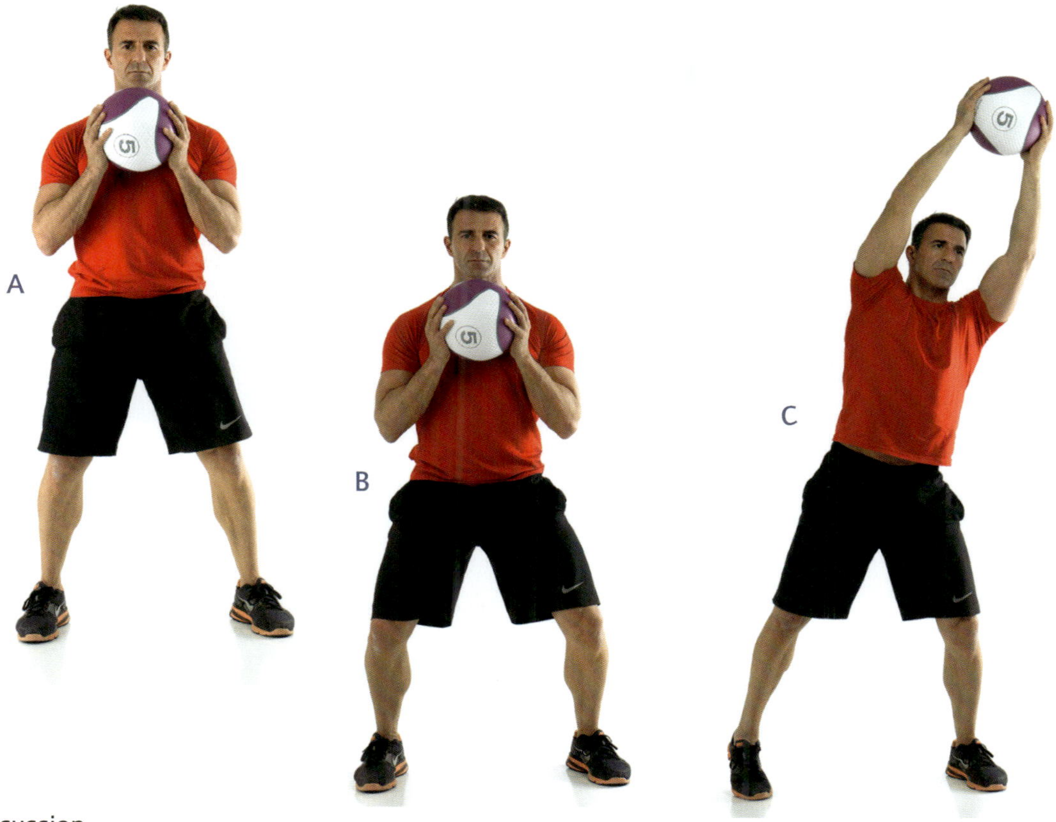

Discussion

The beauty of this truly functional exercise is that people think it is easy. On the contrary, it requires a specific technique which is far from simple. You must imagine you are throwing the med ball from one side to the other; this must be your gesture: to throw, not to lift. Let us analyze the exercise. It is a comprehensive movement. The thrust, quick and explosive, starts from the lower body and involves the hip extensor chain. The movement is then transmitted from the hip to the abdominal fascia

- **D |** Return to center, with the ball at chest height, and execute a quick flexion of the legs again.
- **E |** Now press the ball up diagonally to the right. Complete the required number of repetitions.

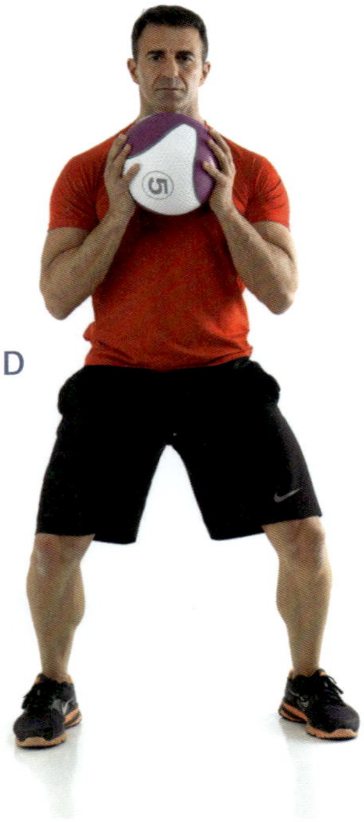
D

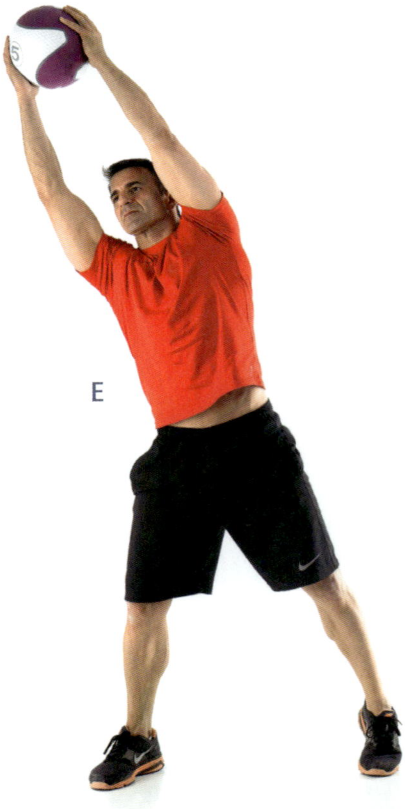
E

and from the core to the upper body, involving the trapezius, deltoid, and triceps. The arm and torso lean, hence the alternate shifting of the weight to the left and right, more heavily involves the contralateral oblique muscles and the ipsilateral deltoid muscle. In other words, when we straighten the arms overhead and to the left, we more heavily involve the torso's right oblique muscles and the left deltoid muscle, and vice versa. Those who haven't practiced multiplanar sporting activities from childhood will struggle, at least initially, when faced with this exercise. All will, however, feel its training value, thanks to the med ball's weight. This is a must in contact sports training.

ONE-ARM BALANCE PRESS

Starting position

- **A |** Stand and hold the medicine ball on the fully-opened palm of the right hand; the ipsilateral arm is close to the side

Execution

- **B |** Extend the right arm up with a controlled movement, lifting the med ball slowly. When you lift a weight above your head with one hand, always look at it. In this case, look toward the med ball.
- **C |** Return back down slowly and complete the set.

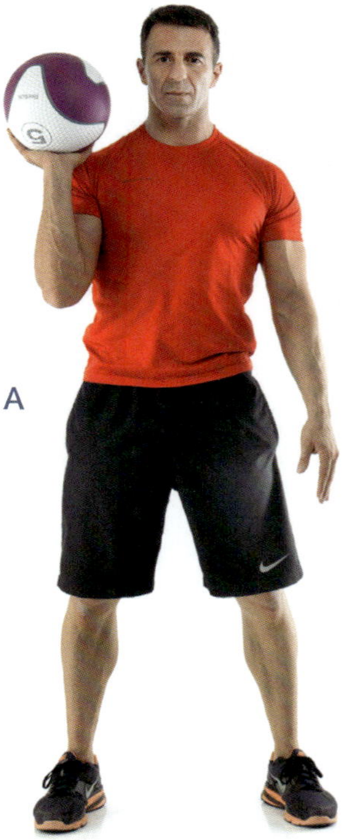

A

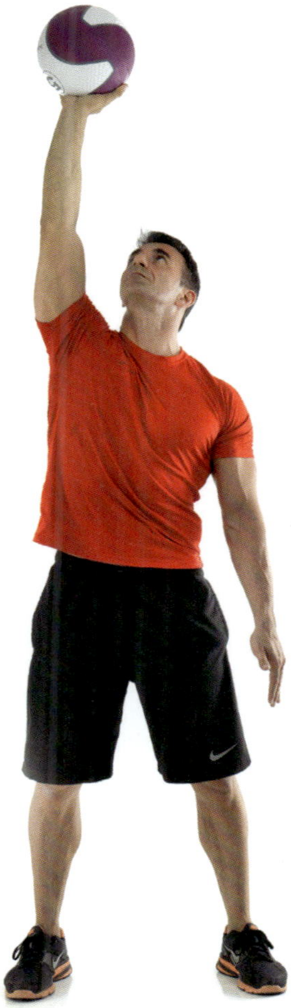

B

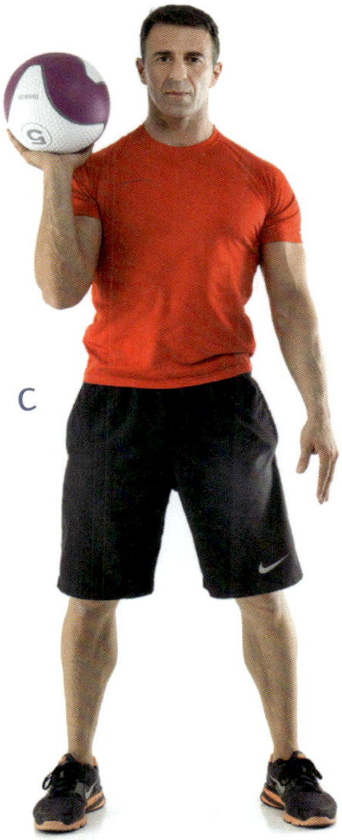

C

- **D and E |** Repeat with the other arm.

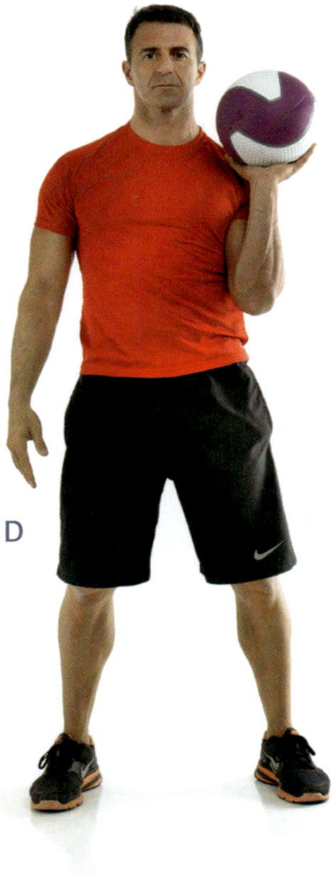

D

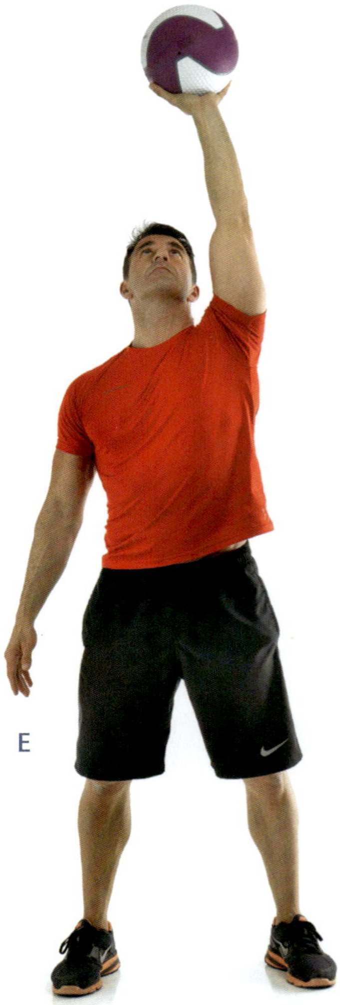

E

Discussion

I realize only now that I haven't talked about balancing exercises yet. They are among my favorites. Few exercises require such movement control, inch by inch. Executing the one-arm balance press you will notice immediately the difference between the right and left arm in terms of strength, coordination, balancing, and individual muscles and how this differential can diminish over time. In fact, balancing exercises allow the control of every single phase of the movement, which can be protracted in time, whittling down the difference between either side of the body, between weak and strong arm, between weak and strong links in the kinematic chains. Balancing exercises are excellent for posture and rehab. Circle it in red and get busy!

TWO-ARM BALANCE PRESS

Starting position

- A | Stand with one med ball in each hand; the palms are open, and the arms are close to the torso.

Execution

- B | Raise the arms up slowly.
Slowly bring them down.
Complete the required repetitions.

A

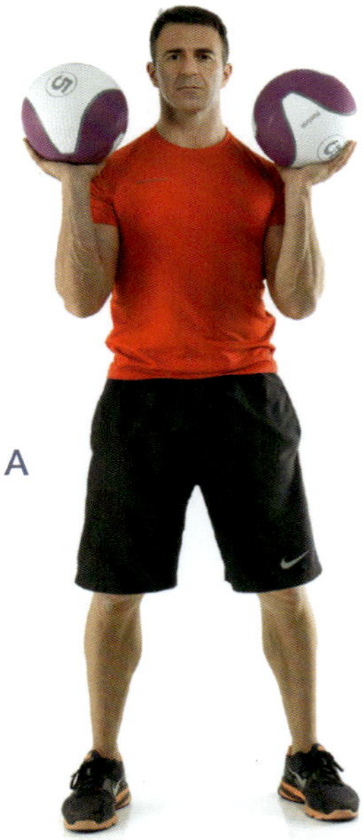

B

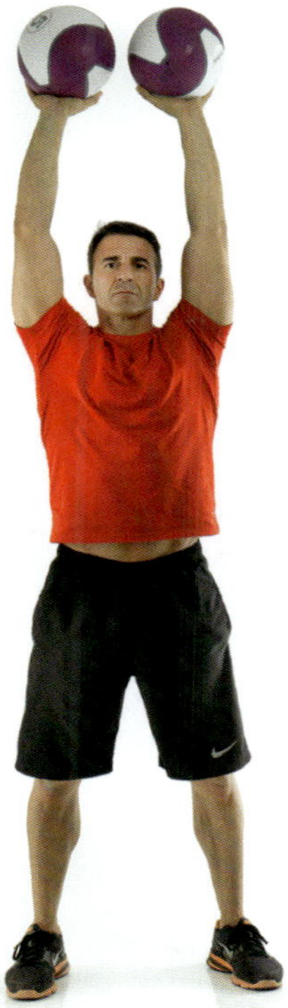

Discussion

A progression of the previous exercise, this is a difficult one, the more so as you increase the med ball's weight gradually as you progress. It provides a good workout not only for shoulders, trapezius, and triceps, but also for the core and the upper pectoralis. It's also excellent training for weak links and stabilizers. Let me repeat it: Balancing exercises are uncommonly comprehensive and unknown in gyms. Yet all sports in which the scapula stabilizers and the rotator cuff are stimulated ought to start from these exercises, for prevention and as an essential part of fitness training.

FRENCH PRESS

Starting position

- A | Lie in the supine position, with the legs bent and the feet resting on the ground. Hold the med ball tight in your hands and lift it above your chest with straight arms.

Execution

- B | Contracting the abdomen slightly to hold the spine's neutral position, flex the arms on the shoulders and slowly bend the elbows until the med ball touches the ground just behind your head. Extending the arms, return to the starting position.

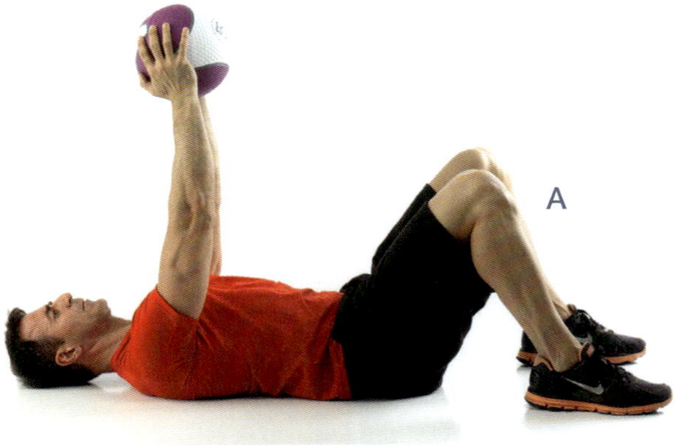

A

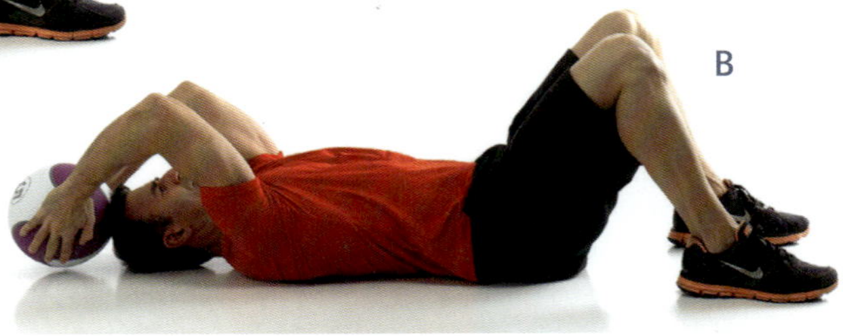

B

Discussion

This is an exercise in which the load has significant importance. The double movement of arm and forearm shouldn't surprise you. Usually in gyms we see the French press executed only by flexing the forearm on the arm, in the eccentric phase, and extending the same in the concentric phase: monoarticular movements therefore, often forgetting the triceps is a muscle with both mono- and biarticular features. The long head both extends and retracts the humerus, besides taking part in the extension of the forearm. Any comprehensive exercise for the triceps must take its biarticularity into account. The French press with med ball isn't a very tough exercise unless executed with significant loads. It can be very interesting for female subjects.

PULL-OVER

Starting position

- **A |** Lie on the ground with the legs bent and feet resting on the floor. Hold the med ball tight in your hands and raise it above your chest with straight arms.

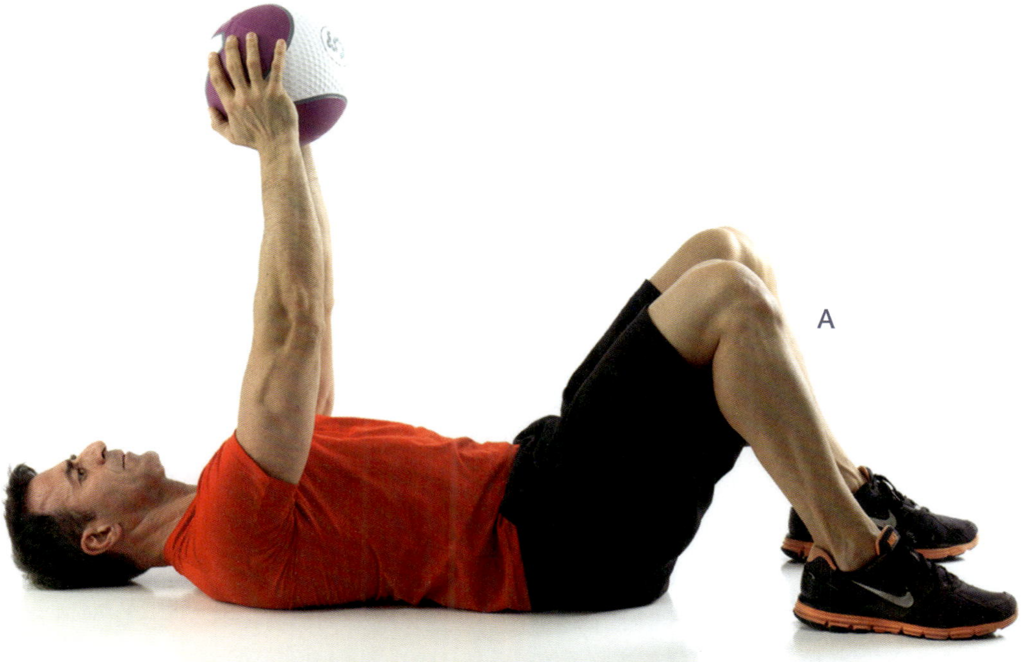

A

Execution

- **B |** Contract the abdomen slightly to hold the spine's neutral position.
  Flex the arms slightly and move the arms slowly backward, until the med ball touches the ground behind you, far from your head. Extend the arms and return to the starting position.

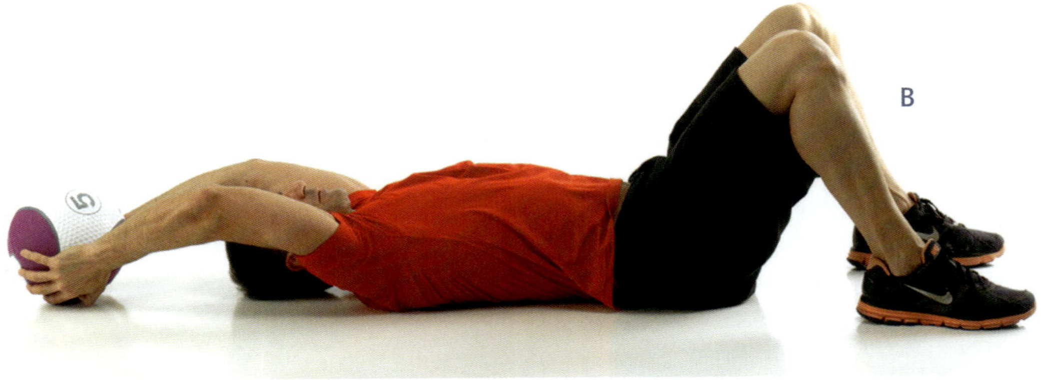

B

Discussion

Let me confess: For a long time I didn't understand the pull-over. All the big guys in the gym did them, but if you asked them what their use was, they replied: "Bah? They work though." In the 1980s it was combined with the respiratory squat as an alternative to crosses, based on the belief—probably true for the under-14s—that it served to increase the volume of the ribcage. You will ask me why I have included it in this book. I could reply "Bah, it works though," but I do have some idea about it. Let's see. The exercise surely stimulates the long head of the triceps, the pectoralis major, latissimus dorsi, and trapezius (and perhaps, I venture a guess, the posterior deltoid). This is quite something: the entire scapulohumeral block. The action of the serratus is actually interesting. This muscle abducts and rotates the scapula externally; together with the rhomboid muscles, it allows the scapula to adhere to the thorax; in particular, it lifts the ribs, because it's a respiratory muscle! Perhaps they were right back in the 1980s?

MED BALL CURL

Starting position

- **A |** Stand with the med ball in your hands; the arms are straight down in front of your torso.

A

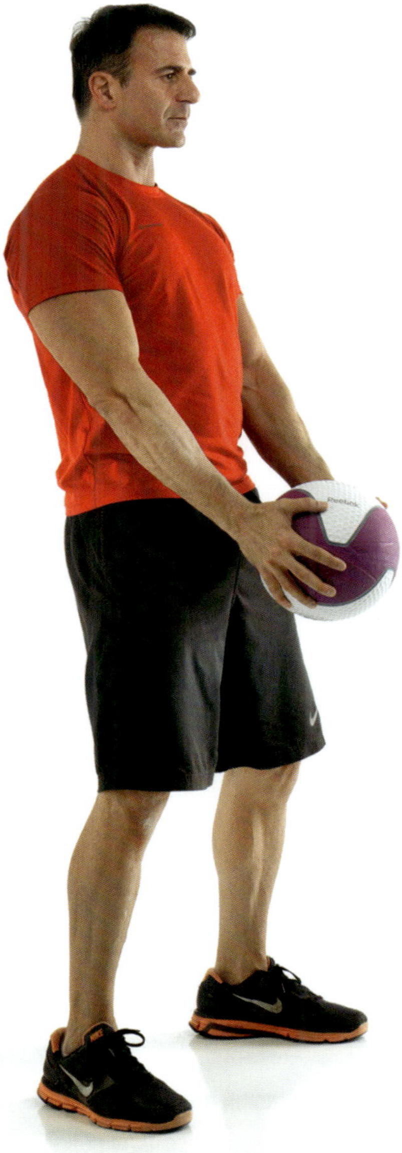

Execution

- **B |** Inhaling, curl up the forearms, bringing the ball toward the chest.
  Flex the arms and slowly return to the starting position
  Complete the required repetitions.

B

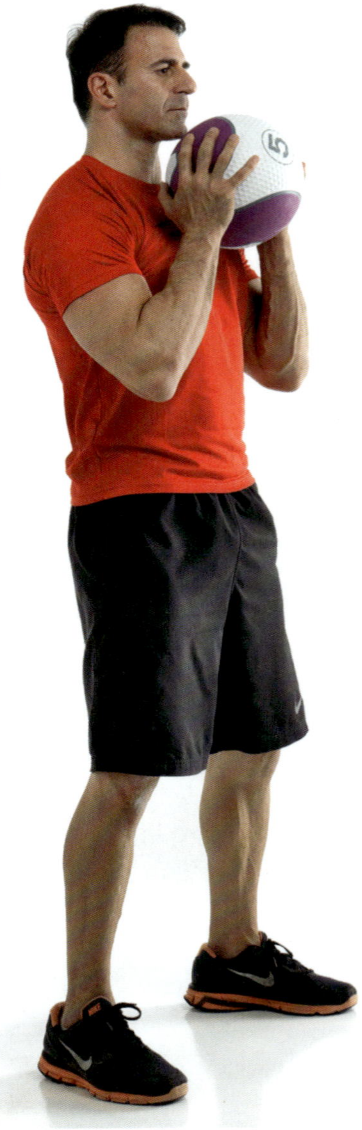

Discussion

The effectiveness of this exercise is influenced significantly by the load used, so by the med ball's weight. What makes it truly interesting compared with a classic barbell or dumbbell curl is the ball's shape, which doesn't allow a stable grip. The med ball's position is guaranteed by the pressure exercised by the arms and transmitted to the hands, and this automatically creates an isometric activation of the pectoralis. This exercise is well-suited for female athletes also those who practice sports in which grip is crucial.

MED BALL SIDE-TO-SIDE HALF-PRESS

Starting position

- A | Stand and bring the ball level with the right shoulder; the right arm is folded and gathered on the side, and the left arm is across the chest, contributing to the med ball's stabilization.

Execution

- B | Raise the right arm and med ball up, bringing the ball just above your head.

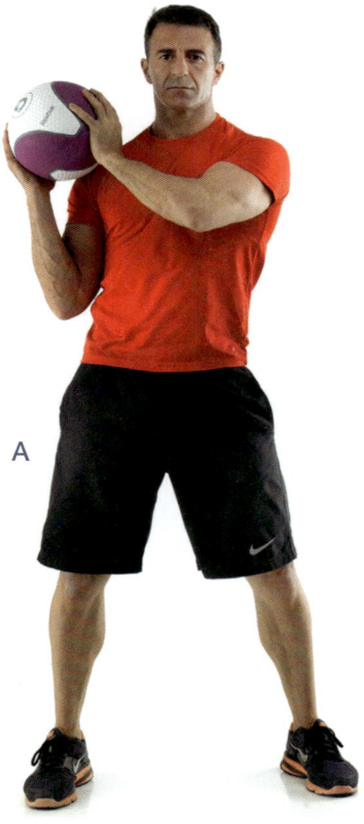

A

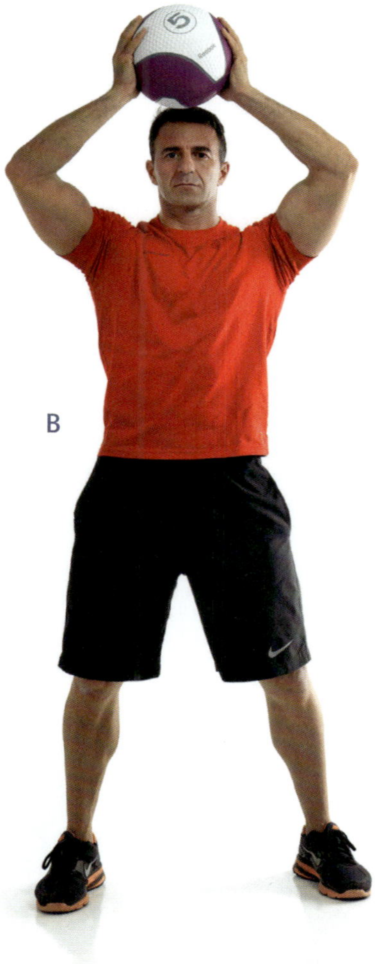

B

Discussion

This is a very intense exercise, especially if performed with a heavy-weight med ball. The arm's abduction, from 0 degrees to 90 degrees and from 90 degrees to 135 degrees, ensures the work depends almost wholly on first the deltoid, and then second the trapezius. The triceps is also involved but to a smaller degree, given that the upward straightening of the arm is halved. The arm which assists

- **C and D |** Return to the starting position but on the opposite side. The left arm takes on the med ball's weight, coming down the same side of the torso; the right arm assists the movement, supporting the left arm. Repeat on the other side. Continue this way, completing the required number of repetitions.

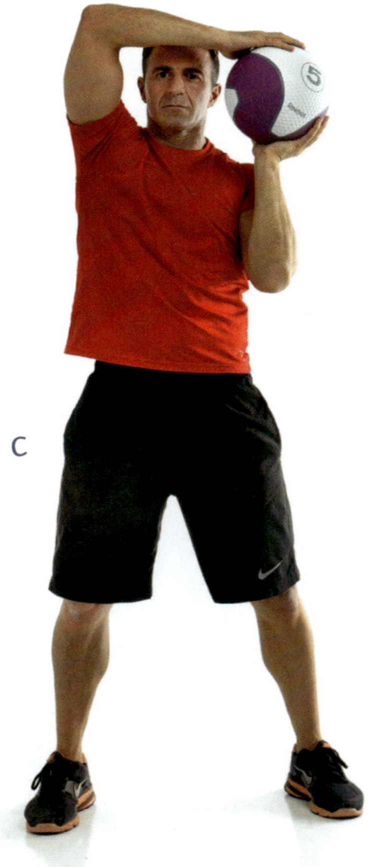

C

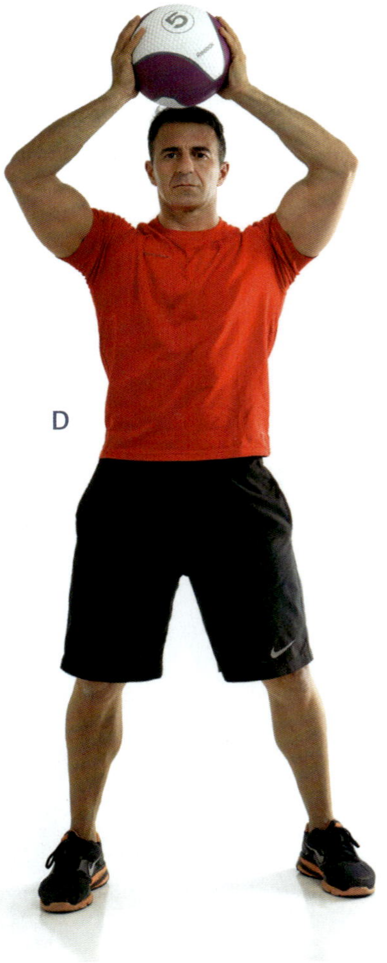

D

the movement by supporting it isn't relaxed, but rather is always slightly raised and flexed frontally. The deltoid muscle works continuously and tires out quickly. This is a significant exercise for training the scapulohumeral girdle, especially for those performance sports (e.g., boxing, combat arts, rugby, and MMA) where this system and the muscles related to it are stimulated in a very intense.

PART III – OBJECTIVES, METHODS, AND TRAINING PROGRAMS

CHAPTER 11

11.1 THE FUNCTIONAL CHOICE

Your body as the best-fitting outfit; a new feeling of efficiency; and technical gestures once unthinkable now become easily-mastered exercises. If you have fully understood the concept of functional training, then maybe you are already feeling all this and experiencing it firsthand. You are only taking your first steps, yet you feel that something is changing, and more will change. I am now forced to dampen your enthusiasm, however, and remind you that functional training is a choice but not an excuse to throw away all you previously practiced in gyms. Actually, its first application is a return to basic exercises, suitably improved and adapted.

Action + Function = Functional training

We must not forget the importance of basic gym exercises such as squats, lunges, pulls, and presses. In this respect, and according to the definition I gave, the performance of weightlifting athletes in clean and jerk and snatch exercises is extremely functional. We have, in fact, an extremely powerful action of the hip extensor chain: a motor action first, then a stabilizing action by the abdominal fascia, and finally, these forces are conducted to the upper body. What do a boxer, a baseball player, a tennis player, and a golfer have in common? Apparently nothing, but if you observe the movement biomechanics, you will find the same concepts previously expressed: wind-up and activation of the hip extensor chain; motor and stabilizing action of the abdominal fascia; and transduction of these forces to the upper body. Have I made myself clear?

The following programs presented in chapters 11 through 13 include bonus exercises which use the following weights: kettlebells, medicine balls, and sandbags. Mastering the exercises in chapter 10 should give you a good foundation for basic form so that if you wish, you can complete the exercises in these programs using various weights. For more details on performing the exercises, see the other volumes in The Ultimate Functional Training Series: *Training With Bodyweight, Training With Kettlebells,* and *Training With Sandbags.*

11.2 STRENGTH TRAINING

We can define strength as the ability to defeat a resistance or to oppose it with a muscular effort (Zatziorskj).

Strength is a conditional ability, which depends about 80% on nerve factors. These factors imply:

- Maximum capacity for recruitment of type II white fibers (IIx especially).
- Maximum development of the central nervous system which, we may remember, takes place approximately by the age of 14.
- The ability to deactivate Renshaw's cells, the cells that act as breakers of the motor message.

The remaining 20% consists of organic and metabolic factors.

- The percentage of type IIa and type IIx white fibers.
- The density, hence the quantity, of white fibers within the transverse section area of the muscle.
- Increase in the diameter of white fibers.
- Improvements in recruitment (see chapter 5).

11.3 STRENGTH-TRAINING PROGRAMS

There are specific programs for strength training. The limit of the programs that follow is that they lack maximal tests and the work on the load percentages for those who pursue such objectives. I have therefore based mine on load progression and on increasing volume and workload by progressively higher-weight percentages within a "wave" program. The positive fact is that they work for everyone.

PROGRAM 1	
WORKOUT A	WORKOUT B
Run 10 min	Run 10 min
Squat 3 x 10.8.6 One-leg kettlebell deadlift 3 x 10 + 10	At-the-shoulder lunge with sandbag 3 x 10 + 10 Overhead squat with kettlebell 3 x 10 + 10
Deadlift 3 x 10.8.6 Pull-up 3 x max	Rower with two sandbags 3 x 10 Clean and press with two kettlebells 3 x 15
Horizontal bench press 3 x 10.8.6 Sandbag clean and press 3 x 15	Front shoulder press with barbell 3 x 10 Snatch with kettlebell 3 x 10
Run 10 min	Run 10 min

Training code
Total-body on major areas
Frequency: 2-3 times per week
Duration: 8-9 weeks
Note to workout A: Rotate the pairs of exercises every week so as to distribute the energies equally on all major areas.
Workout A progression: Every two weeks add a set of 6 to the first exercise in each group with a pyramidal method, up to a maximum of 5
Workout B progression: Every two weeks add 1 set to the first exercise in each listed pair.

PROGRAM 2	
WORKOUT A	**WORKOUT B**
Run 10 min	Run 10 min
Deadlift 4 x 8.6.6.4 Front squat 3 x 10.8.10	One-leg deadlift 3 x 10 One-leg squat 3 x 10
Horizontal bench press 4 x 8.6.6.4 Pull and press with sandbag 3 x 10	Clean and press with sandbag 3 x 20 Sandbag floor pull 3 x 20
Pull-up 4 x max Push press with two kettlebells 3 x 10	Push press with barbell 3 x 10 Tight grip bench 3 x 10
Run 10 min	Run 10 min

Training code
Total-body on major areas
Duration: 8 weeks
Frequency: 3 workouts per week
Notes to sheet A: Rotate the exercise pairs.

PROGRAM 3	
WORKOUT A	**WORKOUT B**
Run 10 min	Run 10 min
Horizontal bench press 5 x 5; recovery 4 min Low pulley 3 x 10; recovery 2 min	Dumbbell press on fitness ball 3 x 10; recovery 1 min 30 sec Clean and press with kettlebell 3 x 10
Squat 5 x 5 Leg curl on fitness ball 3 x 10	Pull-up 3 x max One-leg deadlift with two kettlebells 3 x 10, each side
Deadlift 5 x 5 Lat machine anterior 3 x 10	Barbell curl 3 x 10 Parallel dips 3 x max
Run 10 min	Run 10 min

Training code
Total-body
Duration: 8 weeks
Frequency: 3 times per week

PROGRAM 4	
WORKOUT A	**WORKOUT B**
Run 10 min	Run 10 min
Squat 3 x 7-9; 3 x 4-6; 3 x 11; recovery 4 min	Deadlift 3 x 7-9; 3 x 4-6; 3 x 11
Swing with kettlebell 3 x 20	Floor pull 3 x 20
Military press 3 x 7-9	One-leg deadlift 3 x 7-9
Clean with kettlebell 3 x 20	Walking lunge with rotation 3 x 10, each side
Narrow-grip bench press 3 x 7-9	Barbell curl 3 x 7-9
Run 10 min	Run 10 min
WORKOUT C	
Run 10 min	
Horizontal bench press 3 x 7-9; 3 x 5-7; 3 x 11	
Floor press 3 x 20	
Clean and press with kettlebell 3 x 7-9	
Med ball side lunge with rotation 3 x 10, each side	
Snatch with kettlebell 3 x 20, each side	
Run 10 min	

PROGRAM 5	
WORKOUT A	**WORKOUT B**
Run 10 min	Run 10 min
Power swing with kettlebell 3 x 10 sec	Kneeling jump 3 x 5
Squat 3 x 6; 3 x 3; 3 x 11	Deadlift 3 x 6; 3 x 3; 3 x 9
Pull-up 3 x max	Clean and press with kettlebell 3 x 5-7
Push press with kettlebell 4 x 5-7	One-leg deadlift 3 x 5-7
Barbell curl 3 x 10	Crossover push-up 3 x 10
Run 10 min	Run 10 min
WORKOUT C	
Run 10 min	
Plyo push-up 3 x 5	
Horizontal bench press 3 x 5; 3 x 3; 3 x 9	
Low pulley 3 x 10	
Leopard plank 3 x 20	
Parallel dips 3 x max	
Run 10 min	

CHAPTER 12

12.1 HYPERTROPHY TRAINING

One whole book on this subject wouldn't be enough. There are one thousand and one studies on hypertrophy, but also no certainties as to the mechanism and the cause/effect of the hypertrophic stimulus. Just think about muscular fibers: They can be white, red, intermediate, totipotent, or satellite; each of these responds to one or more different stimuli. Not to mention the other components of the skeletal muscle: the sarcoplasmic, connective or lipid components, or that huge mystery that the brain still is today, with the cerebellum and nervous system, from which everything departs and where everything ends up. This gray area explains the profusion of techniques and methods, ranging from the scientific to the picturesque or the fanciful. Do we have to make do with what is available? Shall we continue with the approximations and anecdotal fantasies of odd guys in gyms? No, we shan't. We must understand our body, a perfect machine to which no computer, even the most advanced, can be remotely compared. Our body has always adapted according to the function for which it was created and has evolved in the course of millennia.

Let's see the priorities then:

1. Training the function of an articular system or a kinematic chain. Do you remember? The purpose, the reason for which that system or chain was built and created and has evolved to the present day.
2. Training the planes involved in the gestures and actions which relate to these systems and kinematic chains. What is the sense of training thighs and glutes with exercises on the frontal plane only (squats and deadlifts) if the hip extensor chain and the coxofemoral joint both share movement ranges on the sagittal and intermediate planes too?
3. Multijoint exercises: There are no monoarticular gestures in daily life.
4. Management and alternation of the loads (i.e., periodization) and the stress induced by them.

This is where I want to start from. I want to integrate an ordinary gym exercise program and its progression with exercises and modifications typical of functional training.

12.2 COSMETIC AND FUNCTIONAL HYPERTROPHY

As I mention in my book *Kettlebell* (Elika Publishers), a dispute is raging in the gym world, a feud which has developed as physical culture has shifted gradually from a performance sport—working on strength and its adaptations—to a sport with purely aesthetic features. The dispute is between cosmetic and functional hypertrophy. Cosmetic hypertrophy, as defined by American athletic coaches, is an increase in muscle mass for its own sake, with the objective of climbing on-stage or exhibiting a well-defined, muscular physique, with no performance purposes. Functional hypertrophy instead is an increase in muscle mass for performance purposes, meaning that it is combined with features such as strength, agility, power, and speed. Where does the main difference between these two cultural extremes lie? In workouts and their adaptations. In workouts we must combine classic basic exercises with functional exercises in order to stimulate different kinematic chains and different motor qualities and skills. As for adaptations, they are connected with functional hypertrophy and involve the central nervous system to a greater degree.

12.3 FUNCTIONAL HYPERTROPHY-TRAINING PROGRAMS

PROGRAM 1	
WORKOUT A	WORKOUT B
Run 8 min	Run 8 min
*Horizontal bench press 3 x 10; recovery 2 min Push-up 3 x max; recovery 1 min 30 sec	*Horizontal bench dumbbell press 3 x 10 Leopard push-up 3 x 10
*Front lat machine (without knee pad) 3 x 10 Floor pull 3 x 10	*Rower with sandbag 3 x 10-15 Lacerta push-up 3 x 10
Barbell push press 3 x 10-12	*Squat jump 3 x 5 Walking lunge & rotation 3 x 5 each side
*Front squat 3 x 10 Walking lunge 3 x 10, each side	Frontal stabilizers on forearms 3 x 10 sec Reverse crunch with sandbag 3 x 10
Straight-arm front stabilizers 3 x 10 sec Oblique crunches 3 x 10, each side	Run 8 min
Run 8 min	

Training code
Total-body
Duration: 6-8 weeks
Progression: every week add 1 set to the exercises marked by *

PROGRAM 2	
WORKOUT A	**WORKOUT B**
Run 8 min	Run 8 min
Horizontal bench press 3 x 10.8.6; recovery 2 min Leopard push-up 3x10, each side; recovery 1 min 30 sec	*Push-up on kettlebells 3 x max Barbell push on fitness ball 3 x 10
Lat machine middle grip (without knee pad) 3 x 10.8.6 Rower with two sandbags 3 x 10, each side	*Sandbag floor pull 3 x 10 Rower with two kettlebells 3 x 10
*Clean and press with two kettlebells 3 x 10 Diagonal press with med ball 3 x 10, each side	Sandbag clean and press 3 x 10
*Front squat with barbell 3 x 10 Walking lunge with rotation 3 x 10, each side	*Squat and press with kettlebell 3 x 10 One-leg kettlebell deadlift 3 x 10, each side
Run 8 min	Side plank with rotation 5 x 10, each side
	Run 8 min

Training code
Total-body
Duration: 6-8 weeks
Progression: every 2 weeks add 1 set to the exercises marked by * (add 1 set of 6 reps to the exercises with pyramidal method)

PROGRAM 3	
WORKOUT A	**WORKOUT B**
Run 8 min	Pull-up 3 x max *Reverse row: horizontal tractions from the multipower bar 3 x max Lacerta push-up 3 x 20
*Front squat 3 x 5 At-the-shoulder lunge with sandbag 3 x 10, each side Power swing 3 x 10	*Double jerk with two kettlebells 3 x 5-7 Diagonal press with med ball 3 x 10, each side Bent press 3 x 7, each side
Plyo push-up 3 x 5-7 *Horizontal bench press 3 x 5 Push-up 3 x 10	Parallel dips 3 x max
Barbell curls from the preacher position (kneeling on a mat, the pelvis off the heels) 3 x 7-9	Leopard plank 3 x 30 sec Reverse rope crunch 3 x 10
Sandbag reverse crunch 3 x 10 Side plank 3 x 10 sec, each side	Run 8 min
Run 8 min	

Training code
Split routine
Duration: 6-8 weeks
Progression: every 2 weeks add 1 set to the exercises marked by *

PROGRAM 4	
WORKOUT A	**WORKOUT B**
Rope skipping 5 min	Run 10 min
Walking lunge with barbell 3 x 5, each side Front squat and press 3 x 7-9 Burpee 3 x 20	Bent press with kettlebell 3 x 7, each side Pull-up 3 x max Sandbag floor pull 3 x 10
Dumbbell push 3 x 5 Leopard push-up 3 x 20	Clean and jerk with two kettlebells 3 x 7 Push press with kettlebell 3 x 15
Narrow-grip bench press 3 x 5	Barbell curl 3 x 5-7
Reverse rope crunch 3 x 20 Side plank with rotation 3 x 10, each side	Leopard plank 3 x 30 sec Side plank with twist 3 x 10, each side
Rope skipping 5 min	Run 10 min

Training code
Split routine
Duration: 6-8 weeks
Progression: every week add 1 set to the first exercise for each muscle group, up to a maximum of 5 sets

CHAPTER 13

13.1 SLIMMING TRAINING

Those who follow me know that slimming is a metabolic condition with several "parents". There are many organic lipolytic paths, meaning there are different methods to start losing body fat. First of all let's clarify what we mean by slimming. We don't simply mean a decrease in weight. Scales are of little use in *slimming* (greatly overweight subjects excepted), because they don't measure the real decrease in body-fat percentage.

How to define slimming then? *Slimming* is a decrease in the lipid organic fractions, especially the subcutaneous and visceral ones. Let me start with a commonplace observation we should, however, keep in mind: There is no slimming without a suitable eating regimen, or at least it is extremely difficult. This point may appear obvious, but it happens to be the basic reason for a lack of results. Having said this, let me be clear that circuit work is suitable for other types of adaptations, too, from hypertrophy to strength. The neurogenic and muscular components involved are determined by the type of training stimulus.

13.2 LIPOLYTIC PATHS

Here is a brief review of the training stimuli to be "administered" (that term isn't chosen at random) to activate different lipolytic paths:

1. Muscle tone training

Muscle tone is a very low-intensity electrical message that is always present in any active muscle, even at rest. This is typically a nerve adaptation, which can be reached by classic strength training. Strength training increases muscle tone over time; this generates an increase in the subject's basal metabolism and an increase in the oxidative work on body fats when at rest, too.

2. Training for hypertrophy

Many people ask me what hypertrophy and slimming have in common. When completing an exercise to exhaustion, lactate production indicates a hormonal response by

- the growth hormone: proteolytic and lipolytic response;
- catecholamines: adrenaline and noradrenalin (lipolytic response); and
- thyroid hormones: lipolytic response.

But is this enough? There is actually more to this; for example, we know that by doing interval work up to the lactate threshold, we influence EPOC heavily. All this translates in a metabolic increase which lasts for several hours after training (depending on the intensity of the exercise, up to 12, 16, even 24 hours and more) with a 10-15% increase in body-fat burning at rest!

3. Aerobic training

The oxidative paths in Krebs cycle are essential in providing the amount of oxygen necessary for lipolysis. Low-intensity aerobic work is indispensable for obese or greatly overweight subjects in the initial phase of training. It is important for beginners, too, though over time the intensity will have to increase progressively, reaching interval training and circuits. Regarding circuits, cardio-fit training, peripheral heart action, and circuit training methods are particularly beneficial.

Further progressions of these are:

- Blitz circuits, for their ability to put all organic systems under heavy stress in a very short time, reaching oxygen debt immediately.
- Timed circuits, for the efficient management of the gesture or gestures being performed.

13.3 CIRCUIT TRAINING

I have been talking about circuit training as the training for the future for at least a decade. You can stimulate highly differentiated systems and organic structures with one single method. Circuit training is essential for general physical preparation for any performance sports-specific training, for strength and hypertrophy training, and for creating a slimming strategy for everyone. The method variations make this a highly diverse type of training, never boring and with a level of intensity ranging from beginners to athletes. The best-known methods are circuit training, cardio-fit training, PHA training, Blitz circuits, timed circuits, and boot camp. Let's take a look at them.

13.3.1 Circuit training

Organized by the US Army around 1956, circuit training consists of a sequence of exercises, varying from 6 to 10 or more, to be repeated with little or no rest between each of them. The execution of one entire sequence of exercises is called a circuit. At the end of each circuit, you can choose between passive or active recovery before starting again.

The number of circuit runs varies from 2 to 10.

PROGRAM 1	PROGRAM 2
TOTAL-BODY PROGRAM FOR EVERYONE	FOR BEGINNER WOMEN
Run 10 min	Run 10 min
Push-up 1 x 10 Crunch 1 x 10 Clean with sandbag 1 x 10 Arms plank 1 x 10 min Walking lunge 1 x 10	Swing with kettlebell 1 x 20 Push-up 1 x 5-10 Walking lunge 1 x 5, 10, each side Arms plank 1 x 10 sec Squat and press with kettlebell 1 x 5/10
Reverse rope crunch 1 x 10 Recovery 2 min	Clean and press with sandbag 1 x 10 Walk 2 min
Repeat the sequence 5 times	Repeat the sequence 3-5 times
Run 10 min	Run 10 sec

PROGRAM 3	PROGRAM 4
FOR BEGINNER MEN	FOR BEGINNER MEN
Run 10 min Push-up 1 x 10 Rope crunch 1 x 10 Floor pull 1 x 10 Forearm plank 1 x 10 sec Front squat 1 x 10 Reverse rope crunch 1 x 10 Rower with sandbag 1 x 10 Leopard plank 1 x 10 sec Recovery 2 min Repeat the sequence 5 times Run 10 min	Run 10 min Leopard plank 1 x 10 Plyo push-up 1 x 5 Reverse rope crunch 1 x 10 Clean and press with kettlebell 1 x 10 Side plank with twist 1 x 10, each side Squat and press with kettlebell 1 x 10 Swing 1 x 20 Recovery 2 min Repeat the sequence 5 times Run 10 min

PROGRAM 5	PROGRAM 6
DYNAMIC EXERCISES FOR BEGINNER WOMEN	DYNAMIC EXERCISES FOR BEGINNER MEN
Run 10 min Jumping jack 1 x 10 Skip 1 x 10 sec Swing 1 x 10 Squat and press 1 x 10 Rope crunch 1 x 10 Push press with kettlebell 1 x 10 Sandbag reverse crunch 1 x 10 Clean and press with sandbag 1 x 10 Recovery 2 min Repeat the sequence 3-5 times Run 10 min	Run 10 min Skip 1 x 10 min Push-up 1 x 10 Jumping jack 1 x 10 Clean and press with sandbag 1 x 10 Burpee 1 x 10 Squat and press with kettlebell 1 x 10 Sandbag reverse crunch 1 x 10 Recovery 2 min Repeat the sequence 3-5 times Run 10 min

PROGRAM 7	PROGRAM 8
FOR INTERMEDIATE MEN	FOR INTERMEDIATE WOMEN
Swing 1 x 20 Leopard push-up 1 x 20 Side plank with twist 1 x 10, each side Burpee 1 x 20 Pull and press with sandbag 1 x 20 At-the-shoulder walking lunge with sandbag 1 x 10, each side Side plank 1 x 10 sec, each side Recovery 2 min Repeat the sequence 5 times Run 10 min	Run 10 min Swing 1 x 20 At-the-shoulder walking lunge with sandbag 1 x 10, each side Clean and press with kettlebell 1 x 10 Swing 1 x 20 Burpee1 x 20 Floor pull 1 x 20 Reverse rope crunch 1 x 20 Push press 1 x 10 Recovery 2 min Repeat the sequence 3-5 times Run 10 min

PROGRAM 9	PROGRAM 10
FOR ADVANCED MEN	FOR ADVANCED WOMEN
Swing 7 min (alternate one-armed and two-armed) Burpee 1 x 20 Push-up with two kettlebells 1 x 20 Med ball side lunge with rotation 1 x 10, each side Leopard plank 1 x 20 Pull-up 1 x 20 Squat and press with kettlebell 1 x 10-20 Rower with sandbag 1 x 20 Side plank with rotation 1 x 5, each side Recovery 2 min Repeat the sequence 5 times Swing 7 min	Swing 7 min Burpee 1 x 20 Leopard plank 1 x 20 Push-up 1 x max At-the-shoulder lunge with rotation 1 x 10, each side Side plank with rotation 1 x 5, each side Clean and press with kettlebell 1 x 10-20 Squat and press with kettlebell 1 x 10 Reverse rope crunch 1 x 20 Rower with sandbag 1 x 20 Recovery 2 min Repeat the sequence 3-5 times Swing 7 min

13.3.2 Cardio-fit training

Cardio-fit training is a circuit training method that alternates aerobic phases—on cardio machines or with aerobic exercises (running, rope skipping, walking)—and anaerobic phases. Initially, the cardio phase is used as active recovery after an exercise phase. The circuit's level of difficulty is increased gradually, heightening the intensity of both the anaerobic and the aerobic phases. Cardio-fit training is a typical interval training method. This is its main strength.

In 1998 it was the subject of a study carried out by Neri, Paoli, and Velussi, who compared its slimming effects to those of the classic method of aerobic training. In the course of the study, they selected two groups of athletes, both composed of beginners. The first group trained on cardio machines only, while the second group performed cardio-fit training with triceps and abs exercises only. The plicometer test results were rather surprising: the degree of slimming in both groups was similar but on triceps and abs the cardio-fit group slimmed down twice as much! At a time when the diatribe on localized slimming was at its peak, the study had a lot of recognition and was the basis for a series of further studies which confirmed its results.

PROGRAM 1	PROGRAM 2
FOR BEGINNER WOMEN	**FOR BEGINNER MEN**
Cardio 10 min	Cardio 10 min
Squat 1 x 5	Push-up 1 x 10
Lateral clean (quadrupedal) 1 x 10, each side	Rope crunch 1 x 10
Repeat 2 times without stopping	Repeat 2-3 times without stopping
Cardio 5 min	Cardio 5 min
Step-up 1 x 5, each side	Squat 1 x 5-7
Backward clean (quadrupedal) 1 x 10, each side	Straight-arm stabilization 1 x 10 sec
Repeat 2 times without stopping	Repeat 2-3 times without stopping
Cardio 5 min	Cardio 5 min
Press with med ball 1 x 10	Press with sandbag 1 x 10
Straight-arm stabilization 1 x 10 sec	Rope diagonal crunch 1 x 5, each side
Repeat 3 times without stopping	Repeat 2-3 times without stopping
Cardio 5 min	Cardio 5 min
Rower with sandbag 1 x 10	Floor pull 1 x 10
Rope crunch 1 x 10	Forearm stabilization 1 x 10 sec
Repeat 3 times without stopping	Repeat 2-3 times without stopping
Cardio 10 min	Cardio 10 min

PROGRAM 3	PROGRAM 4
FOR INTERMEDIATE WOMEN	FOR INTERMEDIATE MEN
Cardio 10 min	Cardio 10 min
Squat jump 1 x 5 Reverse rope crunch 1 x 10 Repeat 3 times without stopping	Med ball crossover push-up 1 x 6, each side Reverse rope crunch 1 x 10 Repeat 3 times without stopping
Cardio 5 min	Cardio 5 min
One-leg kettlebell deadlift 1 x 5, each side Box squat 1 x 5 Repeat 3 times without stopping	Clean and press with sandbag 1 x 10 Side plank with twist 1 x 10, each side Repeat 3 times without stopping
Cardio 5 min	Cardio 5 min
Floor pull 1 x 10 Side plank with twist 1 x 5, each side Repeat 3 times without stopping	Walking lunge 1 x 10, each side Side plank with rotation 1 x 5, each side Repeat 3 times without stopping
Cardio 5 min	Cardio 5 min
Med ball diagonal press 1 x 10, each side Reverse rope crunch 1 x 10 Repeat 3 times without stopping	Rower with two sandbags 1 x 10 Rope diagonal crunch 1 x 10, each side Repeat 3 times without stopping
Cardio 10 min	Cardio 10 min

PROGRAM 5	
FOR ADVANCED WOMEN	
Run 10 min	Cardio 5 min
Kettlebell overhead walking lunge 1 x 10, each side Lateral clean (quadrupedal) 1 x 10, each side Repeat 3 times without stopping	Clean and press with sandbag 1 x 10 Push-up 1 x 10 Repeat 3 times without stopping
Cardio 5 min	Cardio 5 min
Lu.Be.Lu.Be. 1 x 2 rounds, alternating Kettlebell swing 1 x 20 Repeat 3 times without stopping	Floor pull 1 x 15 Side plank with rotation 1 x 5, each side Repeat 3 times without stopping
	Cardio 10 min

PROGRAM 6	
FOR ADVANCED MEN	
Run 10 min Burpee 1 x 10 Leopard crunch 1 x 10, each side Repeat 4 times without stopping Cardio 5 min Sandbag floor pull 1 x 20 Plyo push-up 1 x 7 Repeat 4 times without stopping	Cardio 5 min Clean and press with two kettlebells 1 x 10 Squat and press with two kettlebells 1 x 10 Repeat 4 times without stopping Run 10 min

PROGRAM 7	PROGRAM 8
GENERAL PHYSICAL PREPARATION FOR WOMEN	GENERAL PHYSICAL PREPARATION FOR MEN
Run 10 min Swing 1 x 20 Squat and press with two kettlebells 1 x 10 Repeat 4 times without stopping Cardio 5 min Clean and press with sandbag 1 x 15 Rower with sandbag 1 x 15 Repeat 4 times without stopping Cardio 5 min Push-up 1 x 10 Side plank with rotation 1 x 7, each side Repeat 4 times without stopping Cardio 5 min Burpee 1 x 10 Rope V-crunch 1 x 10, each side Repeat 4 times without stopping Run 10 min	Run 10 min Leopard push-up 1 x 20 Sandbag floor pull 1 x 20 Repeat 4 times without stopping Cardio 3 min Med ball half-kneeling position with rotation 1 x 10, each side Side plank with rotation 1 x 10, each side Repeat 4 times without stopping Cardio 3 min Kettlebell squat and press 1 x 10 One-leg kettlebell deadlift 1 x 10, each side Repeat 4 times without stopping Cardio 3 min Rower with sandbag 1 x 20 Kettlebell renegade row 1 x 10, each side Repeat 4 times without stopping Run 10 min

13.3.3 Peripheral heart action (PHA) training

Created as a bodybuilding technique by Bob Gajda, PHA training has been subsequently applied to circuit training, as a method within the method. It can be applied to all the circuit training programs we have seen so far. It consists of an alternation of selected exercises, working on muscular areas distant from one another.

The distance between the areas stimulates the cardiorespiratory and cardiovascular systems strongly, increasing their activity. Their job is to provide oxygen and metabolites (which are then removed) to the muscles during the exercise. The lipolytic effect is decidedly greater.

Here are some examples of PHA training.

PROGRAM 1	PROGRAM 2
FOR BEGINNER WOMEN	FOR BEGINNER WOMEN
Cardio 10 min Squat 1 x 10 Med ball press 1 x 10 Repeat 3 times without stopping Cardio 5 min Walking lunge 1 x 5, each side Floor pull 1 x 10 Repeat 3 times without stopping Cardio 5 min Push-up with knee support 1 x 5 Rope V-crunch 1 x 5, each side Repeat 3 times without stopping Cardio 5 min Kettlebell swing 1 x 10 Straight-arm plank 1 x 10 sec Repeat 3 times without stopping Cardio 10 min	Cardio 10 min Swing 1 x 20 Squat and press 1 x 10 Repeat 3 times without stopping Cardio 5 min At-the-shoulder walking lunge with sandbag 1 x 10, each side Push-up 1 x 10 Repeat 3 times without stopping Cardio 5 min Kettlebell push press 1 x 10 One-leg kettlebell deadlift 1 x 10, each side Repeat 3 times without stopping Cardio 5 min Rower with sandbag 1 x 15 Reverse rope crunch 1 x 10 Repeat 3 times without stopping Cardio 10 min

PROGRAM 3	PROGRAM 4
FOR BEGINNER MEN	FOR BEGINNER MEN
Cardio 10 min	Cardio 10 min
Squat 1 x 10 Push-up 1 x 10 Repeat 3 times without stopping	At-the-shoulder sandbag squat 1 x 10, each side Med ball crossover push-up 1 x 7, each side Repeat 3 times without stopping
Cardio 5 min	Cardio 5 min
Floor pull 1 x 10 One-leg kettlebell deadlift 1 x 10, each side Repeat 3 times without stopping	Sandbag floor pull 1 x 20 At-the-shoulder sandbag lunge 1 x 10, each side Repeat 3 times without stopping
Cardio 5 min	Cardio 5 min
Med ball diagonal press 1 x 10, each side Plank 1 x 10 sec Repeat 3 times without stopping	Rower with two sandbags 1 x 20 Reverse rope crunch 1 x 15 Repeat 3 times without stopping
Cardio 5 min	Cardio 5 min
Burpee 1 x 5 Rope crunch 1 x 10 Repeat 3 times without stopping	One-leg kettlebell deadlift 1 x 10 Forearm plank 1 x 20 sec Repeat 3 times without stopping
Cardio 10 min	Cardio 10 min

PROGRAM 5	
FOR INTERMEDIATE WOMEN	
Run 10 min	Cardio 5 min
Burpee 1 x 10 Leopard plank 1 x 10, each side Repeat 3 times without stopping	Swing 1 x 30 Reverse rope crunch 1 x 20 Repeat 3 times without stopping
Cardio 5 min	Cardio 5 min
At-the-shoulder sandbag lunge 1 x 10, each side Push-up 1 x 10 Repeat 3 times without stopping	Sandbag floor pull 1 x 20 Med ball diagonal press 1 x 10, each side Repeat 3 times without stopping
	Cardio 10

PROGRAM 6	
FOR INTERMEDIATE MEN	
Run 10 men Swing 1 x 30 Double jerk 1 x 15 Repeat 3 times without stopping Cardio 5 min Kettlebell squat and press 1 x 20 Med ball crossover push-up 1 x 10, each side Repeat 3 times without stopping	Cardio 5 min Sandbag floor pull 1 x 20 Burpee 1 x 20 Repeat 3 times without stopping Cardio 5 min Side plank with twist 1 x 10, each side Kneeling jump 1 x 10 Repeat 3 times without stopping Run 10 min

PROGRAM 7	PROGRAM 8
FOR ADVANCED WOMEN	FOR ADVANCED MEN
Run 10 min Squat and press 1 x 10 Leopard plank 1 x 10, each side Repeat 3 times without stopping Run 5 min Lunge jump 1 x 7, each side Clean and press with sandbag 1 x 20 Repeat 3 times without stopping Run 5 min Squat jump 1 x 5 Plyo push-up 1 x 5 Repeat 3 times without stopping Run 5 min Med ball diagonal press 1 x 10, each side Reverse rope crunch 1 x 15 Repeat 3 times without stopping Run 10 min	Run 10 min Kettlebell squat and press 1 x 20 Leopard plank 1 x 20 Repeat 3 times without stopping Run 5 min Burpee 1 x 20 Leopard push-up 1 x 20 Repeat 3 times without stopping Run 5 min Kneeling jump 1 x 10 Side plank with rotation 1 x 10, each side Repeat 3 times without stopping Run 5 min Sandbag floor pull 1 x 20 Plyo push-up 1 x 10 Repeat 3 times without stopping Run 10 min

13.3.4 Blitz circuits

Widespread test evidence suggests we should bear in mind the following factors as the keys to reaching different objectives.

SLIMMING

1. Gradual work on EPOC is essential; increases in EPOC are related to the intensity of the exercise rather than its duration.
2. Increase in metabolic "horse power" through an increase in lean mass; the lean mass increase is chiefly promoted by lactacid work.
3. Muscle tone work; muscle tone increase (a much underestimated concept) is connected to alactacid training.
4. Lipolytic hormones activation (GH, testosterone, catecholamines, thyroid hormones) through lactacid-alactacid work.

TONING

1. Lean mass increase.
2. Muscle tone increase.
3. Anabolic hormones activation (GH, IGF-1, IGF-2, testosterone, FGF, insulin) through lactacid-alactacid work.
4. Training should concentrate exclusively on alactacid-lactacid workouts.

Starting from these premises I have developed blitz training circuits that are fast, intense, and effective. They last up to 30 min, and this is more than enough! Blitz circuit effectiveness is related to its intensity; basic exercise selection will be key, as well as the loads, which will point in the direction of the desired objective (slimming, toning, muscle tone, or hypertrophy).

PROGRAM 1	PROGRAM 2
SLIMMING	**SLIMMING FOR WOMEN**
Cardio 5 min: ideally walking, (stationary) steps, running, horizontal bike Dynamic deadlift 1 x 15 Rower with barbell 1 x 15 Front squat 1 x 15 Front shoulder press 1 x 15 Repeat 3-5 times without stopping Cardio 5 min **Note:** The barbell must be the same light weight for all the exercises in the circuit. The subject will pick up the barbell at the start of the blitz and will not set it down until the end of the workout.	Cardio 5 min: ideally walking, (stationary) steps, running, horizontal bike Front squat 1 x 10 Rower with barbell 1 x 15 Walking lunge 1 x 5, each side Front shoulder press 1 x 15 Repeat 3-5 times without stopping Cardio 10 min **Note:** The execution should not be too quick. It is important to find your own cadence and rhythm and to maintain it, improving gradually.

PROGRAM 3	PROGRAM 4
TONING	**ATHLETIC TRAINING**
Cardio 5 min: ideally walking, (stationary) steps, running, horizontal bike Squat 1 x 10 Front shoulder press 1 x 10 Walking lunge 1 x 10, each side Bar tractions (dips) 1 x 10 Repeat 5 times without stopping Cardio 5 min **Note:** Once you have grasped the blitz concept, it is important to move beyond these outlines and adapt them to our clients. Blitz circuits are extremely versatile and can be adapted to any subject, even beginners, by fine-tuning loads and intensity.	Running or rope skipping 5 min Power swing (very heavy load) 1 x 10 Horizontal bench press 1 x 5 Power swing 1 x 10 Squat 1 x 5 Power swing 1 x 10 Chin-ups 1 x 5-7 Repeat 3-5 times without stopping Cardio 5 min

PROGRAM 5	PROGRAM 6
FOR FEMALE SUBJECT WITH CELLULITE OR OTHER CIRCULATORY PROBLEMS	**FOR MMA**
Cardio 8 min Swing 1 x 10 Push-up 1 x 10 Front squat 1 x 5 Rower with sandbag 1 x 10 Step-up (two steps) 1 x 5, each side Repeat 3-5 times without stopping Cardio 8 min	Rope skipping 8 min Kettlebell clean and press 1 x 15 Burpee 1 x 10 Kettlebell squat and press 1 x 15 Bar pull-up 1 x max Med ball lunge with rotation 1 x 10, each side Push-up 1 x 15 Repeat 5-10 times without stopping Rope skipping 8 min
Note: The swing must be executed fast but with a rather light load. Load the front squat with 8 RM. The step-up exercise is essential to work on plantar arch circulation and help the venous blood flow.	**Note:** Plan a mini-recovery at the end of each circuit. Question: How long does a MMA bout last for? You will have to continue working non-stop on the circuit for the same amount of time. From here on, managing your energy levels throughout the bout will not be a problem.

PROGRAM 7	PROGRAM 8
GENERAL PHYSICAL PREPARATION	**GENERAL PHYSICAL PREPARATION FOR WOMEN**
Cardio 10 min Kettlebell squat and press 1 x 15 Sandbag snatch 1 x 10 Med ball diagonal press 1 x 10, each side Crossover lunge 1 x 10, each side Rower with sandbag 1 x 20 Side plank with twist 1 x 10, each side Repeat 5-10 times without stopping Cardio 10 min	Cardio 10 min Kettlebell power swing 1 x 10 At-the-shoulder sandbag squat 1 x 10, each side Floor pull 1 x 20 One-leg kettlebell deadlift 1 x 10, each side Push-up 1 x 10 Repeat 5-10 times without stopping Cardio 10 min

13.3.5 Timed circuits

The timed circuit concept was inspired by kettlebell work. In this type of circuit training you don't count sets and reps but only work for the preset time. You can apply this methodology, fine-tuning the exercises and the repetitions, on any type of subject: sedentary, intermediate, advanced, or athletes. You can also manage intensity (i.e., the effort expended in each single set), exercise by exercise, according to the student's degree of fitness and his or her special needs. Since the objective is long-duration work, managing the right level of intensity is clearly of utmost importance. For this reason I suggest starting with a load of about 10 RM, with only 5-6 reps per set.

PROGRAM 1	
ANTI-CELLULITE	
Uphill walking 15 min (3% slope; 2.8-3.1 mi/h [4.5-5 km/h]) Coreboard step-up 1 x 5, each leg Quadruped backward leg lift 1 x 10, each leg	Leg curl with fitness ball 1 x 5 Swing with kettlebell 1 x 10 Repeat for 10-20 min without stopping Uphill walking 15 min (3% slope; 2.5 mi/h [4 km/h])
Note: If the subject is a beginner, you will start with a 5-min workout, gradually increasing the time with each workout. Execution throughout the circuits will have to be extremely careful to maximize the training stimulus. The versatility of timed circuits and circuit training in general makes for virtually infinite combinations.	

PROGRAM 2	
MULTI-DISTRICT WOMAN	
Uphill walking 10 min (3% slope; 2.8-3.1 mi/h [4.5-5 km/h]) Kettlebell or dumbbell swing 1 x 15 Quadruped backward leg lift 1 x 10, each leg Step-up on two steps 1 x 5, each leg Straight-leg quadruped lateral lunges 1 x 5, each leg Repeat for 10 min without stopping Cardio 5 min or active recovery 3 min Plank stabilization 1 x 20 sec Oblique crunches 1 x 5, each side	Lateral stabilization 1 x 15 sec, each side Reverse crunch 1 x 5 Repeat for 10 min without stopping Cardio 5 min Push press with dumbbells 1 x 6 Renegade row 1 x 5, each side Push-up 1 x 6 Floor pull 1 x 6 Repeat for 10 min without stopping Walking 10 min (cool-down)

PROGRAM 3	
TOTAL BODY	
Walking 10 min (warm-up) Front squat 1 x 5 Floor pull 1 x 6 Walking lunge 1 x 5, each leg Push press with kettlebell 1 x 6 Repeat for 10 min without stopping Cardio 5 min Sandbag pull and press 1 x 6 Push-up 1 x 6 Rower with sandbag 1 x 6	Frontal stabilization 1 x 20 sec Repeat for 10 min without stopping Cardio 5 min Kettlebell clean and press 1 x 6 Oblique rope crunches 1 x 10, each side Swing with kettlebell 1 x 15 Reverse rope crunch 1 x 10 Repeat for 10 min without stopping Walking (cool-down) 10 min
Note: Timed circuit training for advanced subjects marks the evolution from sportsperson to athlete; it forces you to refine your technique—your energy management and economy of gestures on the one hand and reduction of risks and increase in benefits on the other.	

PROGRAM 4	
FOR THE INTERMEDIATE ATHLETE	
Run 10 min Horizontal bench press 1 x 6 Front squat 1 x 6 Low pulley 1 x 6 One-leg kettlebell deadlift 1 x 5, each side Repeat for 10 min without stopping Active recovery 3 min or cardio 5 min Kettlebell push press 1 x 6 Rower with sandbag 1 x 6	At-the-shoulder sandbag lunge 1 x 6 Med ball burpee 1 x 6 Repeat for 10 min without stopping Active recovery 3 min Kettlebell swing 1 x 10 Plyo push-up 1 x 5 Kettlebell deadlift 1 x 6 Sandbag floor pull 1 x 6 Repeat for 10 min without stopping Cardio 10 min

13.3.6 Boot camps

Boot camp training is a circuit training method based on the military courses used by soldiers worldwide for their operational training. It reached Italy, riding the popularity wave of training methods such as cross-fit and kettlebell training. It is an excellent, engaging group workout system. Boot camp training features a great variety in terms of exercise setting, exercise equipment, training intensity, and the management of groups ranging in numbers from 10 people to several hundreds. Boot camp training relies on the coach's ability in setting the course, planning the sequence and duration of exercises, and on the enthusiasm of fitness lovers ready to work out anywhere, whether in a park or a garage. I will never forget my experience at the summer 2012 boot camp in San Diego, California for the IDEA World Convention.

Warm-up: a 4 km (2.5 mi) run to the USS Midway aircraft carrier, moored in San Diego harbor. One hour of intense body-weight exercises led by Todd Durkin and his staff, then another 4-km cool-down run back to the San Diego Convention Center. Coming back to us, how can you set up a functional boot camp in a gym? This is actually rather simple. A lot depends on the number of people involved and the method used.

We shall therefore distinguish different approaches, based on a different number of stations according to how many the participants are. There are essentially three variables in this kind of circuit training:

1. the exercises
2. the exercise execution time
3. the recovery time between each station

The **exercises** must be extremely simple, especially for beginners and in each boot camp's initial circuits.

Execution time varies with each exercise. What does it depend on? On the objectives of the people you are training. Are you dealing with a group of athletes practicing lactacid or mixed sports (with energy delivery lasting from 30 sec and up)? Workout time will be 30-40 sec per station (as training progresses, you may increase this).

Are you dealing with a group of athletes practicing alactacid sports (power, expressions of strength, and explosiveness for 5-20 sec) ? Plan stations of 10-20 sec, up to a maximum of 30 sec. What about beginners, fitness lovers, and subjects with no competitive yearnings? Start with simple exercises lasting a maximum of 20 sec.

Moving from one station to another will be the circuit's active recovery time. This will have to be carefully measured out according to the subjects you are training. With athletes, the time can be progressively shortened, from 20 sec or less. You can actually turn the transfer from one station to another into an exercise; for example, you can reach the next station in a walking lunge, leopard plank, or leopard push-up. With beginners or occasional gym patrons, recovery time should definitely be higher. If the workout time at the station is, for example, 20 sec, recovery time between stations should be at least 30 sec. The last factor is space. The limit of an indoor boot camp is the space available. This is why I will restrict my indications to the number of people statistically more likely, given the usual size of gyms.

2 BOOT CAMP STATIONS	
Groups between 8 and 20 people	
Split the people into two distinct groups: Group 1 and Group 2. Group 1 (G1) will do a standing body-weight workout. Group 2 (G2) will work on mats. Assign an exercise to both groups. Execution time: Begin with 20 sec per station. Warm-up time: 10 min.	
Circuit 1 G1: squat 1 x 20 sec G2: crunch 1 x 20 sec Switch the exercises and repeat. Repeat this pair of exercises three times per group, with a 20-sec recovery time between exercises.	**Circuit 3** G1: floor pull 1 x 20 sec G2: reverse crunch 1 x 20 sec Switch the exercises and repeat. Repeat this pair of exercises three times per group, with a 20-sec recovery time between exercises.
Circuit 2 G1: Walking lunge 1 x 20 sec G2: arm stabilization 1 x 20 sec Switch the exercises and repeat. Repeat this pair of exercises three times per group, with a 20-sec recovery time between exercises.	**Circuit 4** G1: leopard push-up G2: forearm stabilization 1 x 20 sec Switch the exercises and repeat. Repeat this pair of exercises three times per group, with a 20-sec recovery time between exercises.

4 BOOT CAMP STATIONS

Groups between 16 and 40 people

Split the participants into four groups:
G1, G2, G3, G4.
Set up four exercise stations: A, B, C, D.

Assign a muscle area to each station:

A = dynamic legs
B = core training
C = classic legs
D = trunk and upper body

Develop four exercises per station.

A
- Jumping jack
- Skip
- Starter
- Burpee

B
- Crunch
- Straight-arm plank
- Reverse crunch
- Plank with twist

C
- Squat
- Walking lunge
- Crab
- Lunge with rotation

D
- Push-up
- Lacerta push-up
- Leopard push-up
- Floor pull

Rules

1. Assign one group per station.
2. Assign and demonstrate to each group the first exercise in each station (Jumping jack, crunch, squat, push-up).
3. Start the clock: 20 sec to execute the maximum number of reps.
4. After 20 sec, stop the exercise and signal the station change.
5. Each group has 20 sec to transfer to the next exercise station.
6. Start the clock again for another 20 sec.
7. Repeat the sequence so that each group will complete the four stations circuit (Jumping jack, crunch, squat, push-up) three times.
8. Now pause so that athletes can recover and drink some water; then show each group the second exercise in each station (skip, straight-arm plank, walking lunge, lacerta push-up)
9. Start the cycle again, completing four circuits, with three sets per exercise.

ETHICS AND CONCLUSIONS

If you have come this far, then probably you are in it up to your neck... like me. Functional training improves your mind and body, makes you more open and observant, and, makes you a better person (why not?).

Your body will become a perfectly tailored outfit, your mind always lucid, and your senses focused to the max. You will enjoy your training and every moment of your life with an intensity you have never experienced before.

If you have come this far, please read these last few lines.

ETHICS OF THE FUNCTIONAL ATHLETE

1. Train by using your body.
2. Keep your eyes open, watch and discover new exercises.
3. Always keep your mind open.
4. Continue along your course: Improvement has no limits.
5. Compare your method, you will find certainties.
6. Love who you are and what you do.

Happy training, everybody!

CREDITS

Cover design: Kristina Ehrhardt, Anja Elsen

Cover photos: © Guido Bruscia and Thinkstock/iStock

Photos: Chapter images on p. 18, 19 32, 33, 35, 44, 45, 64, 80, 91, 111: Shutterstock (www.shutterstock.com)
Chapter graphics: © Thinkstock/iStock

Layout: Kristina Ehrhardt, Anja Elsen

Typesetting: www.satzstudio-hilger.de

Copyediting: Elizabeth Evans

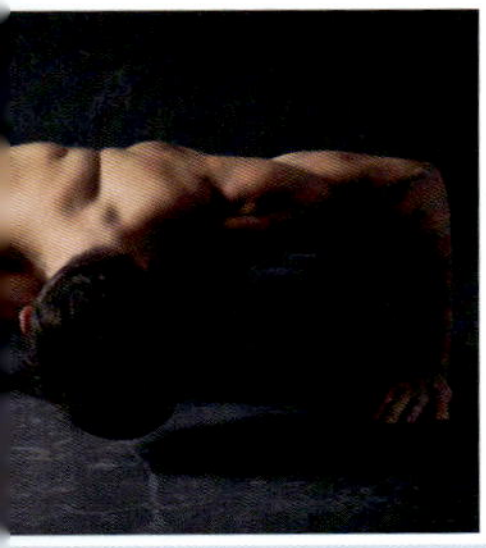

THE ULTIMATE FUNCTIONAL

OUT DECEMBER 2024

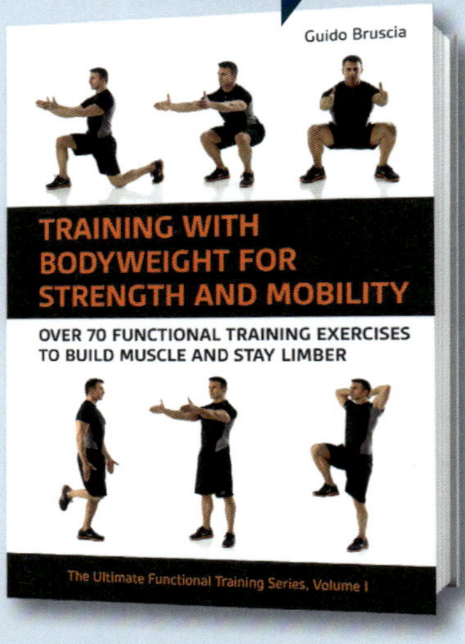

Volume I

ISBN 978-1-78255-273-4

$26.95 US

OUT APRIL 2025

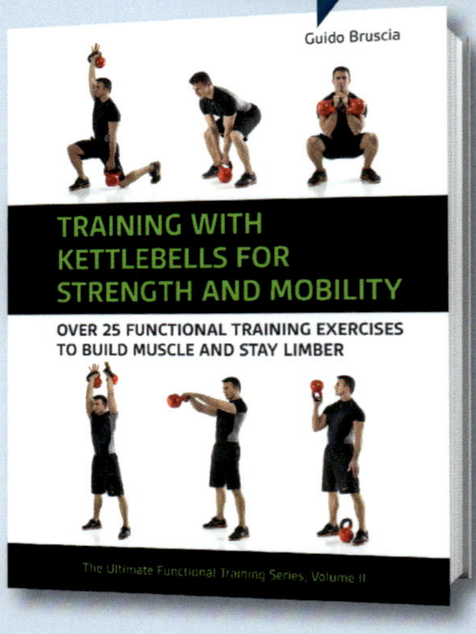

Volume II

ISBN 978-1-78255-283-3

$24.95 US

MEYER & MEYER SPORT

MEYER & MEYER Sport
Von-Coels-Str. 390
52080 Aachen
Germany

Phone +49 02 41 - 9 58 10 - 13
Fax +49 02 41 - 9 58 10 - 10
E-Mail sales@m-m-sports.com
Website www.m-m-sports.com

TRAINING SERIES

IN FOUR VOLUMES!

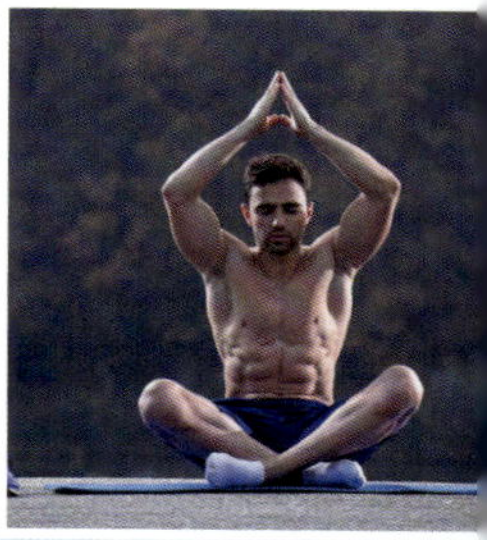

OUT OCTOBER 2025

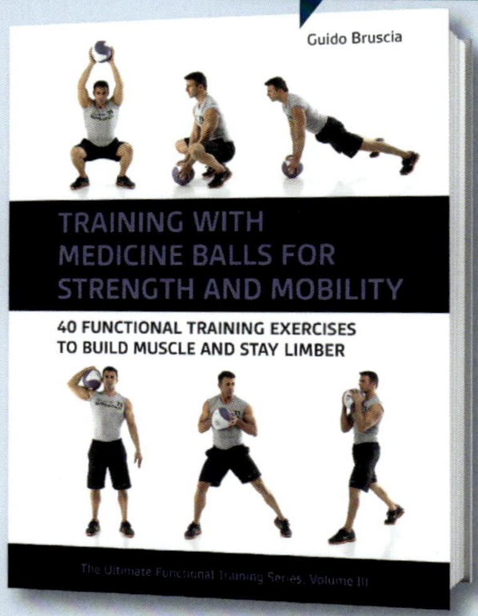

Volume III

ISBN 978-1-78255-289-5

$26.95 US

OUT MARCH 2026

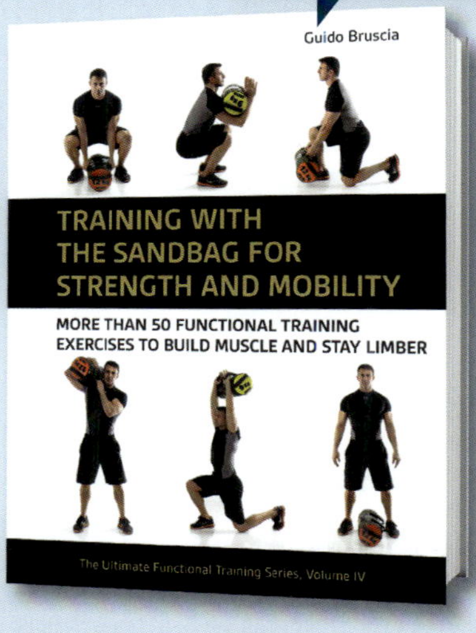

Volume IV

ISBN 978-1-78255-292-5

$26.95 US

MEYER & MEYER Sport
Von-Coels-Str. 390
52080 Aachen
Germany

Phone +49 02 41 - 9 58 10 - 13
Fax +49 02 41 - 9 58 10 - 10
E-Mail sales@m-m-sports.com
Website www.m-m-sports.com

MEYER & MEYER SPORT

MEYER & MEYER HAS THE BEST IN FITNESS & STRENGTH TRAINING!

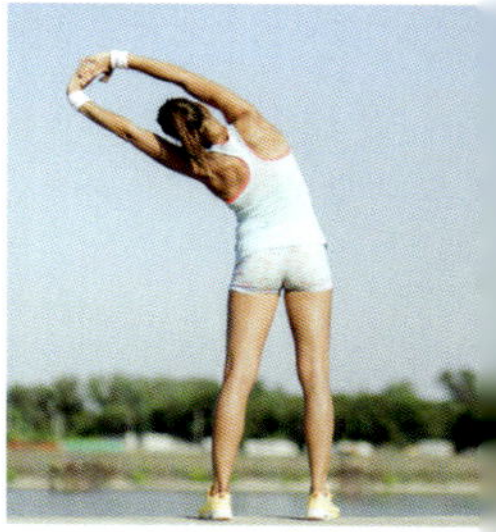

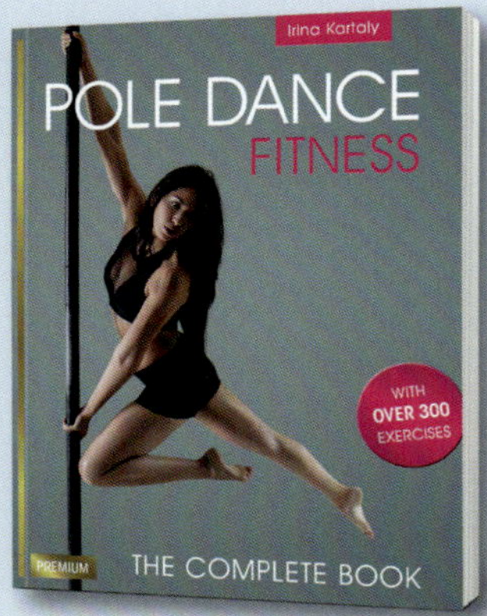

ISBN 9781782551935
$22.95 US

INCLUDES DEMO VIDEOS!

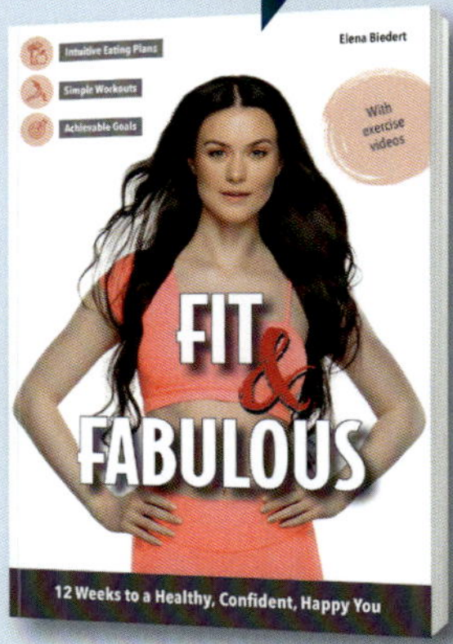

ISBN 9781782552086
$24.95 US

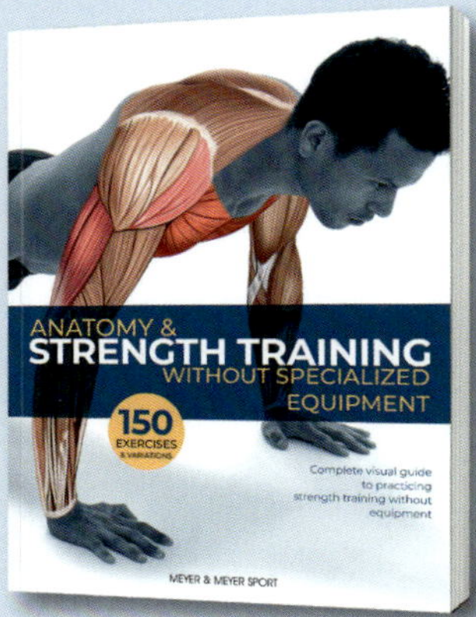

ISBN 9781782551935
$22.95 US

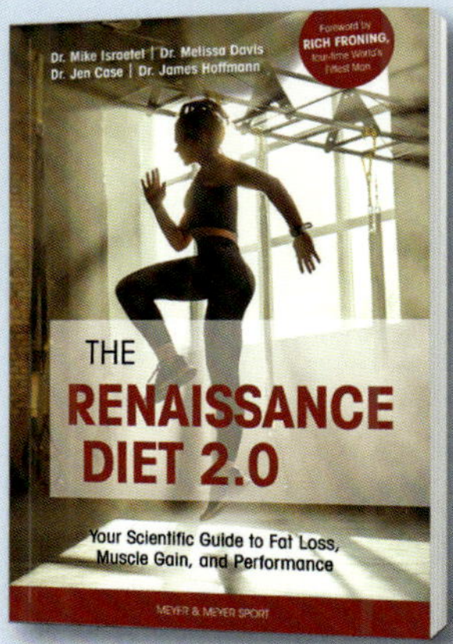

ISBN 9781782551904
$26.95 US

MEYER & MEYER Sport
Von-Coels-Str. 390
52080 Aachen
Germany

Phone +49 02 41 - 9 58 10 - 13
Fax +49 02 41 - 9 58 10 - 10
E-Mail sales@m-m-sports.com
Website www.m-m-sports.com

MEYER & MEYER SPORT